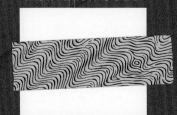

Surgery for Urinary Incontinence

FEMALE PELVIC SURGERY VIDEO ATLAS SERIES
Series Editor:

Mickey Karram, MD
Director of Urogynecology
The Christ Hospital
Clinical Professor of Obstetrics and Gynecology
University of Cincinnati
Cincinnati, Ohio

Other Volumes in the Female Pelvic Surgery Video Atlas Series

Basic, Advanced, and Robotic Laparoscopic Surgery
Tommaso Falcone & Jeffrey M. Goldberg, Editors

Hysterectomy for Benign Disease
Mark D. Walters & Matthew D. Barber, Editors

Management of Acute Obstetric Emergencies
Baha M. Sibai, Editor

Posterior Pelvic Floor Abnormalities
Tracy L. Hull, Editor

Surgical Management of Pelvic Organ Prolapse
Mickey Karram & Christopher Maher, Editors

Urologic Surgery for the Gynecologist and Urogynecologist
John B. Gebhart, Editor

Vaginal Surgery for the Urologist
Victor Nitti, Editor

FEMALE PELVIC SURGERY VIDEO ATLAS SERIES
Mickey Karram, Series Editor

Surgery for Urinary Incontinence

Roger Dmochowski, MD

Professor of Urology
Director, Pelvic Medicine and Reconstruction Fellowship
Department of Urology
Professor of Obstetrics and Gynecology
Vice Chair, Section of Surgical Services
Vanderbilt University Medical Center;
Executive Medical Director for Patient Safety and Quality (Surgery)
Associate Chief of Staff
Medical Director of Risk Management
Vanderbilt University Hospital
Nashville, Tennessee

Mickey Karram, MD

Director of Urogynecology
The Christ Hospital;
Clinical Professor of Obstetrics and Gynecology
University of Cincinnati
Cincinnati, Ohio

W. Stuart Reynolds, MD, MPH

Assistant Professor
Female Pelvic Medicine and Reconstructive Surgery
Department of Urologic Surgery
Vanderbilt University Medical Center
Nashville, Tennessee

Illustrated by **Joe Chovan, Milford, Ohio**

ELSEVIER
SAUNDERS

1600 John F. Kennedy Blvd.
Ste 1800
Philadelphia, PA 19103-2899

SURGERY FOR URINARY INCONTINENCE   ISBN: 978-1-4160-6267-7

Notices

Knowledge and best practice in this field are constantly changing. As new research and experience broaden our understanding, changes in research methods, professional practices, or medical treatment may become necessary.

Practitioners and researchers must always rely on their own experience and knowledge in evaluating and using any information, methods, compounds, or experiments described herein. In using such information or methods they should be mindful of their own safety and the safety of others, including parties for whom they have a professional responsibility.

With respect to any drug or pharmaceutical products identified, readers are advised to check the most current information provided (i) on procedures featured or (ii) by the manufacturer of each product to be administered, to verify the recommended dose or formula, the method and duration of administration, and contraindications. It is the responsibility of practitioners, relying on their own experience and knowledge of their patients, to make diagnoses, to determine dosages and the best treatment for each individual patient, and to take all appropriate safety precautions.

To the fullest extent of the law, neither the Publisher nor the authors, contributors, or editors, assume any liability for any injury and/or damage to persons or property as a matter of products liability, negligence or otherwise, or from any use or operation of any methods, products, instructions, or ideas contained in the material herein.

Library of Congress Cataloging-in-Publication Data

Dmochowski, Roger R.
  Surgery for urinary incontinence / Roger Dmochowski, Mickey Karram, W. Stuart Reynolds; illustrated by Joe Chovan.
      p. ; cm.—(Female pelvic surgery video atlas series)
  Includes bibliographical references and index.
  ISBN 978-1-4160-6267-7 (hardcover : alk. paper)
  I. Karram, Mickey M.   II. Reynolds, W. Stuart (William Stuart)   III. Title.   IV. Series: Female pelvic surgery video atlas series.
    [DNLM: 1. Urinary Incontinence—surgery—Atlases.   2. Postoperative Care—methods—Atlases.   3. Postoperative Complications—prevention & control—Atlases.   4. Treatment Outcome—Atlases.   5. Urologic Surgical Procedures—methods—Atlases. WJ 17]
    616.6'2—dc23

                                                                    2012049117

Senior Content Strategist: Stefanie Jewell-Thomas
Senior Content Development Specialist: Arlene Chappelle
Content Development Manager: Maureen Iannuzzi
Publishing Services Manager: Deborah L. Vogel
Senior Project Manager/Project Manager: Jodi M. Willard/Kamatchi Madhavan
Design Direction: Lou Forgione

Last digit is the print number: 9   8   7   6   5   4   3   2   1

This book is dedicated to my parents, Leon and Sheila Dmochowski, for providing me the ability to complete an education in a free country. To my wife, Suzanne, who has been supportive over many long years of academic turbulence. It is also dedicated to my sons, Nick and Colin, who have given me great pleasure and who are the light of my life. Finally, I would like to dedicate this book to my two mentors in urology, Dr. Herbert Seybold and Dr. Joseph Corriere. Both of these giants of Texas urology provided me with the impetus to begin a career in what has turned out to be a very fulfilling avocation, that being urology.

—Roger Dmochowski

To my father, Herbert Reynolds, MD, for his legacy of medical professionalism and dedication to academic and scientific progress; and to my mother, Anne Reynolds, for her unwavering support and enthusiasm for even the smallest of successes.

To my wife, Carolyn, and daughters, Emma and Sarah, for their support and patience and for inspiring me to strive to improve the experience of pelvic floor disorders in women of all ages.

—W. Stuart Reynolds

This book is dedicated to my mentors. I have been very fortunate to have been guided professionally and academically by a number of individuals who unselfishly provided me education and opportunities that significantly impacted my professional and academic careers in a very positive way. I strive to provide the same type of guidance and support to the various individuals that I have the luxury of mentoring.

—Mickey Karram

Contributors

Roger Dmochowski, MD
Professor of Urology
Director, Pelvic Medicine and Reconstruction Fellowship
Department of Urology
Professor of Obstetrics and Gynecology
Vice Chair, Section of Surgical Sciences
Vanderbilt University Medical Center;
Executive Medical Director for Patient Safety and Quality (Surgery)
Associate Chief of Staff
Medical Director of Risk Management
Vanderbilt University Hospital
Nashville, Tennessee
1: Etiology and Epidemiology of Urinary Incontinence; 2: Preoperative Evaluation of Patients with Urinary Incontinence and Selection of Appropriate Surgical Procedures for Stress Incontinence; 5: Biologic Bladder Neck Pubovaginal Slings; 6: Retropubic Synthetic Midurethral Slings; 8: Single-Incision Synthetic Midurethral Slings; 9: Surgical Management of Voiding Dysfunction and Retention After Stress Incontinence Surgery; 10: Bulk-Enhancing Agents for Stress Incontinence: Indications and Techniques; 11: Sacral Neuromodulation; 12: Botulinum Toxin Injection Therapy; 13: Bladder Augmentation; 14: Mixed and Recurrent Incontinence, Incontinence in Patients with Pelvic Organ Prolapse, and How Best to Avoid and Manage Complications: Case Discussions

Mickey Karram, MD
Director of Urogynecology
The Christ Hospital
Clinical Professor of Obstetrics and Gynecology
University of Cincinnati
Cincinnati, Ohio
2: Preoperative Evaluation of Patients with Urinary Incontinence and Selection of Appropriate Surgical Procedures for Stress Incontinence; 3: Surgical Anatomy of the Anterior Vaginal Wall, Retropubic Space, and Inner Groin; 5: Biologic Bladder Neck Pubovaginal Slings; 6: Retropubic Synthetic Midurethral Slings; 7: Transobturator Synthetic Midurethral Slings; 8: Single-Incision Synthetic Midurethral Slings; 9: Surgical Management of Voiding Dysfunction and Retention After Stress Incontinence Surgery; 14: Mixed and Recurrent Incontinence, Incontinence in Patients with Pelvic Organ Prolapse, and How Best to Avoid and Manage Complications: Case Discussions

Melissa R. Kaufman, MD
Assistant Professor
Department of Urologic Surgery
Vanderbilt University Medical Center
Nashville, Tennessee
1: Etiology and Epidemiology of Urinary Incontinence; 5: Biologic Bladder Neck Pubovaginal Slings; 6: Retropubic Synthetic Midurethral Slings; 10: Bulk-Enhancing Agents for Stress Incontinence: Indications and Techniques; 11: Sacral Neuromodulation; 12: Botulinum Toxin Injection Therapy; 13: Bladder Augmentation

W. Stuart Reynolds, MD, MPH
Assistant Professor
Female Pelvic Medicine and Reconstructive Surgery
Department of Urologic Surgery
Vanderbilt University Medical Center
Nashville, Tennessee
1: Etiology and Epidemiology of Urinary Incontinence; 2: Preoperative Evaluation of Patients with Urinary Incontinence and Selection of Appropriate Surgical Procedures for Stress Incontinence; 5: Biologic Bladder Neck Pubovaginal Slings; 6: Retropubic Synthetic Midurethral Slings; 8: Single-Incision Synthetic Midurethral Slings; 10: Bulk-Enhancing Agents for Stress Incontinence: Indications and Techniques; 11: Sacral Neuromodulation; 12: Botulinum Toxin Injection Therapy; 13: Bladder Augmentation; 14: Mixed and Recurrent Incontinence, Incontinence in Patients with Pelvic Organ Prolapse, and How Best to Avoid and Manage Complications: Case Discussions

Mark D. Walters, MD
Professor and Vice Chair of Gynecology
Department of Obstetrics and Gynecology
Obstetrics, Gynecology, and Women's Health Institute
Cleveland Clinic
Cleveland, Ohio
4: Retropubic Operations for Stress Urinary Incontinence

Dani Zoorob, MD
Urogynecology Fellow
The Christ Hospital
University of Cincinnati
Cincinnati, Ohio
5: Biologic Bladder Neck Pubovaginal Slings; 6: Retropubic Synthetic Midurethral Slings; 7: Transobturator Synthetic Midurethral Slings; 8: Single-Incision Synthetic Midurethral Slings

Video Contributors

Rodney A. Appell, MD, FACS†
Formerly Director, Texas Continence Center
Vanguard Urologic Institute
Memorial Hermann Texas Medical Center
Houston, Texas
Video: *Cystoscopic Injection of Urethral Bulking Agent (Coaptite)*

Elizabeth Graul, MD
Phase II Women's Center
Salt Lake City, Utah
Video: *Cystoscopic Injection of Urethral Bulking Agent (Coaptite)*

Vincent R. Lucente, MD, MBA, FACOG
Medical Director, Institute for Female Pelvic Medicine and Reconstructive
Surgery;
Medical Director, FPM Urogynecology Center;
Chief, Gynecology, St Luke's University Health Network;
Clinical Professor, ObGyn
Temple University
Philadelphia, Pennsylvania
Video: *AJUST Adjustable Single-Incision Sling*

Ayman Mahdy, MD, PhD
Assistant Professor of Urology
Director of Voiding Dysfunction and Female Urology
Department of Surgery, Division of Urology
University of Cincinnati College of Medicine
Cincinnati, Ohio
Video: *Technique for Bladder Augmentation (Example 2)*

Harout Margossian, MD
Assistant Clinical Professor
Downstate University Medical School;
Director, Urogynecology Department Ob/Gyn
Lutheran Medical Center
Brooklyn, New York
Video: *Laparoscopic Paravaginal Repair*

Tristi Muir, MD, FACOG
Associate Professor
Departments of Obstetrics and Gynecology and Urology
Medical Director, Pelvic Health and Continence Clinic
Obstetrics and Gynecology
University of Texas Medical Branch
Galveston, Texas
Video: *Vaginal Urethrolysis*

Marie Fidela R. Paraiso, MD, FACOG
Professor of Surgery
Section Head, Urogynecology and Reconstruction Pelvic Surgery
Obstetrics and Gynecology and Women's Health Institute
The Cleveland Clinic
Cleveland, Ohio
Video: *Laparoscopic Paravaginal Repair*

Mary South, MD, FACOG
Assistant Professor
Director, Division of Female Pelvic Medicine and Reconstructive Surgery
Department of Obstetrics and Gynecology
University of Cincinnati College of Medicine
Cincinnati, Ohio
Video: *Technique for Bladder Augmentation (Example 2)*

James L. Whiteside, MD, MA, FACOG
Co-Director of Female Pelvic Medicine and Reconstructive Surgery
The Christ Hospital
Cincinnati, Ohio
Video: *Anatomy Relevant to Transobturator Midurethral Slings*

Preface

"The important thing is not to stop questioning. Curiosity has its own reason for existing."
"Insanity is doing the same thing over and over again but expecting different results."
"Not everything that counts can be counted and not everything that can be counted counts."

—Albert Einstein

These three quotes by Albert Einstein allude to the philosophies that should guide us in the surgical management of women with urinary incontinence.

These various procedures continue to evolve in light of emergent technologies and an aging female population. The demand and real societal need for successful management options for urinary incontinence are critical because the impact of this condition on women's lives and productivity is substantive.

As of yet, there is no one management solution that addresses stress, urge, or mixed incontinence definitively. New technologies have come forward that attempt to address these conditions in minimally invasive and therapeutic fashions; however, the common coexistence of multiple symptoms related to stress incontinence and overactive bladder makes durable and definitive solutions with single interventions rarely applicable. There continues to be a real need to understand the appropriate indications, use of new technologies, and management of complications related to both older and newer type interventions for incontinence in women. The answer when a procedure has failed is not to repeat the same intervention repetitively but to thoughtfully seek the reason for failure and have sufficient experience in alternatives in order to create a strategy that provides the maximum potential benefit to the patient.

This volume is one of an eight-part book series known as "Female Pelvic Surgery Video Atlas Series." The goal of this book is to present a technical guide for procedures and interventions for urethral sphincteric incontinence as well as incontinence resulting from detrusor compliance abnormalities. The procedures discussed and demonstrated are the ones most commonly used for these conditions and have been demonstrated to have efficacy, durability, and safety in the extant medical evidence base. Illustrations and videos serve as additional exemplars for technique and approach. The authors would like to commend and recognize illustrator Joe Chovan, as well as the video contributors as delineated in the frontispiece.

This volume is meant to be comprehensive yet objective, presenting the nuances of appropriate preoperative preparation and postoperative management. This textbook also addresses management of complications, which can be extremely detrimental to long-term functional outcomes related to both standard and newer techniques.

The book begins with a review of the etiology and epidemiology of urinary incontinence. Chapter 2 is a detailed review of the preparation for patients with all types of urinary incontinence and the selection of the appropriate interventions for the diagnosed type of incontinence. Chapter 3 provides an anatomic demonstration of the anterior vaginal wall, retropubic space, and inner groin for the purpose of understanding the aspects of the anatomy pertinent to the interventions discussed. Chapter 4 details the standard retropubic operations for urinary incontinence, including both the Burch and paravaginal repairs. Chapter 5 discusses and demonstrates bladder neck biologic pubovaginal slings and the associated aspects of tissue harvest or tissue selection. Chapter 6 begins a series of chapters dealing with synthetic midurethral slings. Chapter 6 deals with specifically retropubic midurethral slings, Chapter 7 details the transobturator route, and Chapter 8 discusses single-incision slings. Inherent in all of these discussions is a review of the factors of selection as well as the specifics of operative technique conducive to optimal outcome. Chapter 9 summarizes the management of voiding dysfunction and retention after all types of anti-incontinence procedures. Chapter 10 assesses the current status of bulking agents, specifically techniques for implantation. Chapters 11 to 13 discuss surgical interventions for detrusor compliance abnormalities, specifically, sacral nerve stimulation, botulinum toxin therapy, and bladder augmentation. The final chapter concludes with an overview of the management of mixed incontinence and incontinence associated with pelvic organ prolapse and how best to avoid and manage complications related to the various procedures for stress incontinence.

We hope that this text, with the visual aids of the illustrations and video clips, provide all levels of surgeons—including practitioners, residents, and fellows in training—with the most recent advancements in surgical procedures to correct urinary incontinence in women. Implicit in all of these interventions is a well-informed and counseled patient. Although our ability to understand each individual's goal for therapy has improved from even a few years ago, every woman has individual desires, fears, and concepts about her condition that the provider must recognize and assuage. Individualized and realistic goal setting is critical to satisfaction. Time and compassion are as important as surgical intervention and provide the foundation for successful management of this condition.

Roger Dmochowski, MD
Mickey Karram, MD
W. Stuart Reynolds, MD, MPH

Contents

10 Bulk-Enhancing Agents for Stress Incontinence: Indications and Techniques 127

Roger Dmochowski, MD, W. Stuart Reynolds, MD, and Melissa R. Kaufman, MD

Video Demonstration

11 Sacral Neuromodulation 135

W. Stuart Reynolds, MD, Melissa R. Kaufman, MD, and Roger Dmochowski, MD

Video Demonstrations

12 Botulinum Toxin Injection Therapy 153

W. Stuart Reynolds, MD, Melissa R. Kaufman, MD, and Roger Dmochowski, MD

Video Demonstration

13 Bladder Augmentation 161

W. Stuart Reynolds, MD, Melissa R. Kaufman, MD, and Roger Dmochowski, MD

Video Demonstrations

14 Mixed and Recurrent Incontinence, Incontinence in Patients with Pelvic Organ Prolapse, and How Best to Avoid and Manage Complications: Case Discussions 169

Mickey Karram, MD, W. Stuart Reynolds, MD, and Roger Dmochowski, MD

Video Demonstrations

Etiology and Epidemiology of Urinary Incontinence

1

W. Stuart Reynolds, M.D.
Melissa R. Kaufman, M.D.
Roger Dmochowski, M.D.

Introduction and Definitions

Urinary incontinence (UI), according to the International Continence Society (Haylen et al., 2010), is defined as the involuntary loss of urine. It simultaneously exists as a symptom or complaint, sign, or finding and defined condition. Within the broad context of lower urinary tract symptoms (LUTS), UI is considered a storage symptom as opposed to a voiding symptom: "storage" refers to the filling phase of the micturition cycle, whereas "voiding" refers to the emptying phase.

The most commonly recognized subtypes of UI are stress urinary incontinence (SUI), urge urinary incontinence (UUI), and mixed urinary incontinence (MUI). SUI is the involuntary loss of urine associated with effort or physical exertion (e.g., sporting activities) or sneezing or coughing. UUI is the involuntary loss of urine associated with urgency, a sudden, compelling desire to pass urine that is difficult to defer. MUI is a combination of the former two—the involuntary loss of urine associated with urgency and with effort or physical exertion or sneezing or coughing. Other types of UI include functional UI, related to inability to reach the toilet in an otherwise normal urinary system; overflow UI, resulting from bladder overdistention or retention; and enuresis, insensible and continuous incontinence.

Symptoms and findings of UI often coexist with other, associated LUTS, including symptoms related to storage and voiding. Overactive bladder (OAB) syndrome is the constellation of multiple storage symptoms predicated by urinary urgency, usually accompanied by frequency and nocturia, with or without UUI, in the absence of urinary tract infection (UTI) or other obvious pathology. Frequency, urgency, and nocturia can also occur separately. Voiding symptoms that may coexist with UI include hesitancy, slow or weak urinary stream, straining to void, incomplete bladder emptying, dysuria, and retention. Pain, either specific to pelvic organs (e.g., bladder, urethra, vaginal, rectal/anal) or generalized, can also occur.

Voiding dysfunction is a diagnosis made on the basis of symptoms and clinical findings and defined as abnormally slow or incomplete micturition, including acute or chronic urinary retention. It most typically occurs in women as an adverse outcome after invasive treatment for SUI or other pelvic floor conditions.

UI and LUTS often occur in women in association with other pelvic floor conditions, including pelvic organ prolapse (POP). SUI is commonly found in women with POP, although as the degree of POP increases, SUI becomes less apparent, and other LUTS may develop. Often SUI can be demonstrated in this scenario by reducing the POP and testing for SUI. When SUI is observed only after the reduction of coexistent prolapse, it is referred to as occult or potential SUI.

Epidemiology and Economic Impact

UI is a common condition in women. Estimates vary by definition, but approximately 25% to 75% of women report some UI. In the United States, approximately half of surveyed women report some UI, whereas 16% report UI of at least moderate severity. Projections of prevalence based on population growth suggest that the number of U.S. women with UI will increase by more than 50% (from 18 million to 28 million women) from 2010 to 2050. Minassian et al. (2008) reported that 23% to 38% of the female population in the United States older than age 20 admit to symptoms of SUI. It is estimated that 7% to 10% of women affected perceive SUI as being severe with frequent leakage (Thom et al., 2005). Analysis of Medicare data suggests that only approximately 10% of women diagnosed with SUI undergo surgical correction (Anger et al., 2009).

SUI is the most common subtype of UI reported by women: about 50% of women with UI report SUI as the primary or sole symptom of incontinence. About one third of women with UI have MUI, and 15% have UUI alone. Concurrent POP or fecal incontinence or both are common, occurring in 23% of women with UI. Even when UI is recognized, a substantial number of women do not receive a formal diagnosis or do not seek treatment. Of women with no prior diagnosis of UI, 50% report some degree of urine leakage.

Age and race/ethnicity directly affect prevalence estimates. The prevalence of SUI increases with age initially, peaks around the fourth or fifth decade, and then decreases with increasing age. In contrast, MUI and UUI generally increase with age, eventually overtaking SUI by the sixth or seventh decade. SUI is more common in white and Hispanic women than black women; UUI may be more common in black women.

Longitudinal data estimate the risk of developing any UI can be 40%, with an annual incidence of 3% to 11%. In middle-aged women, SUI most commonly develops. Annual incidence of SUI is estimated to be 4% to 11%, and remission is estimated to be 4% to 5% per year. As mentioned, as age increases, the risk of MUI and UUI increase, whereas the risk of SUI decreases.

Although all subtypes of UI represent a significant burden to individuals and health care systems, SUI is the subtype that is most amenable to surgical treatment. It was estimated that 12% of U.S. women underwent SUI surgery in 2003; future projections suggest this will increase by almost 50% over the next 40 years (from 200,000 in 2010 to 300,000 in 2050). A woman born in the United States has a lifetime risk of 11% of undergoing a surgical procedure for incontinence or prolapse by the age of 80.

The economic impact of UI and pelvic floor conditions is significant. Pelvic floor disorders accounted for 4 million ambulatory outpatient visits in 2006 in the United States, with an estimated cost of $412 million. In 1995, annual direct costs for UI in women in the United States were $12.4 billion. Individually, women with UI spend up to $900 a year for routine care, including protective pads and laundry services. Women seeking surgical treatment for SUI paid $118 per month for complete resolution of UI. Increased costs are particularly pronounced for women older than age 65, and Medicare spending continues to increase substantially for treatment of UI. For OAB syndrome, estimates for the

U.S. population suggest $65 billion is spent annually on direct and indirect costs, with projections for 2020 of $82 billion.

Etiology and Risk Factors

Etiology of Urinary Incontinence

The pathophysiology underlying UI is often multifactorial and specific to the subtype of UI (i.e., SUI vs. UUI). In UUI, detrusor overactivity or involuntary bladder contraction is the etiologic event that results in the incontinence episode. Causes for detrusor overactivity are varied and include neurologic injury (brain or spinal cord); changes to lower urinary tract function owing to aging, hormone withdrawal, or bladder outlet obstruction; or, in most cases, idiopathic causes.

Neurologic injury typically results in the loss of voluntary control of voiding, which leads to an uncoordinated OAB (neurogenic bladder). For lesions of the cerebral cortex or basal ganglia (i.e., suprapontine), damage to the brain induces overactivity by reducing voluntary inhibition of voiding, while typically preserving sensation and coordination of the sphincter. For lesions below the brainstem, including the spinal cord, damage eliminates voluntary and coordinated control of voiding, resulting in detrusor overactivity mediated by spinal reflex pathways. Typically, loss of bladder sensation occurs, as does coordination between detrusor contraction and urinary sphincter relaxation (i.e., detrusor-sphincter dyssynergia). Neurologic damage to structures distal to the spinal cord, including nerve roots or peripheral nerves, also can result in bladder and lower urinary tract dysfunction. Crush injury to the pudendal nerve during labor and delivery is thought to contribute to SUI. Systemic conditions, such as multiple sclerosis, can affect multiple components of the neurologic pathways, resulting in varied voiding abnormalities (Table 1-1).

In nonneurogenic situations, including idiopathic, detrusor overactivity can develop as a result of pathophysiologic changes to the bladder muscle, affecting contractility, and to the balance between motor and sensory innervation. The effects of age, hormone withdrawal, bladder outlet obstruction, local hypoxia, or partial denervation on the bladder tend to promote detrusor contraction and overactivity. Hypersensitivity or oversensitivity of the afferent (i.e., sensory) nerves of the bladder may also trigger detrusor overactivity.

For SUI, the mechanisms are different: changes to anatomic support, structural components, and function of the urethra and bladder neck contribute primarily to incontinence episodes. Factors in part necessary for maintenance of urinary continence and prevention of urinary loss include a healthy,

Table 1–1 Common neurologic conditions affecting bladder function and the lower urinary tract

Brain	Spinal Cord	Peripheral Nerves
Cerebrovascular disease (stroke)	Multiple sclerosis	Vertebral disk disease
Traumatic brain injury	Spinal cord injury	Spinal stenosis
Dementia	Cervical myopathy	Radical pelvic surgery
Cerebral palsy	Acute transverse myelitis	Herpesvirus (zoster)
Parkinson disease	Neurospinal dysraphism	Diabetes mellitus
Brain tumor	Tabes dorsalis, pernicious anemia	Guillain-Barré syndrome
Cerebellar ataxia	Poliomyelitis	Trauma (labor/delivery)
Multiple system atrophy		

Table 1–2 Potential risk factors associated with stress urinary incontinence

Age*	Hysterectomy
Parity*	Physical activity
Vaginal delivery*	Smoking
Obesity/BMI*	Diet
Diabetes*	Other medical conditions
Hormone replacement therapy*	Family history*

BMI, Body mass index.
*Factors consistently associated with increased risk.

functioning striated sphincter; well-vascularized urethral submucosal tissue; and intact vaginal wall support. When any of these factors are compromised, the urethra may not remain closed at rest or during increased abdominal pressure, and SUI ensues. Loss of vaginal or pelvic floor support to the urethra and bladder allows the urethra to "sag" inappropriately during periods of increased abdominal pressure (i.e., stress or strain): the proximal urethra rotates and descends away from its retropubic position. Urethral closure is prevented, and urinary leakage occurs. This change in urethral position is commonly described as hypermobility. Primary urethral sphincter weakness independent of hypermobility (i.e., intrinsic sphincter deficiency) can also result in SUI. In this situation, coaptation of the urethral mucosa is lost, as a result of deficient sphincter mass or function or submucosal tissue cushions or both. Traditionally, intrinsic sphincter deficiency and urethral hypermobility were viewed as dichotomous mechanisms for SUI; however, current understanding of the pathophysiology of SUI assigns these factors to a mechanistic continuum, whereby most women have a component of both factors.

Risk Factors

Multiple risk factors have been proposed and studied for the development of SUI in women. SUI is a multifactorial health condition with many contributing factors involved in the pathogenesis. Table 1-2 lists potential risk factors that have been more widely studied. Among those listed, age, parity, vaginal delivery, obesity and body mass index, hormone replacement, diabetes, and family history have been reproducibly associated with increased risk of SUI across most studies.

Suggested Readings

Anger JT, Weinberg AE, Albo ME, et al. Trends in surgical management of stress urinary incontinence among female Medicare beneficiaries. *Urology.* 2009;74:283-287.

Fowler CJ, Griffiths D, de Groat WC. The neural control of micturition. *Nat Rev Neurosci.* 2008;9: 453-466.

Haylen BT, De Ridder D, Freeman RM, et al. An International Urogynecological Association (IUGA)/ International Continence Society (ICS) joint report on the terminology for female pelvic floor dysfunction. *Neurourol Urodyn.* 2010;29:4-20.

Koelbl H, Nitti V, Baessler K, Salvatore S, Sultan A, Yamaguchi O. Pathophysiology of urinary incontinence, faecal incontinence and pelvic organ prolapse. *Incontinence.* 2009;4:255-330.

Minassian VA, Stewart WF, Wood GC. Urinary incontinence in women: variation in prevalence estimates and risk factors. *Obstet Gynecol.* 2008;111(2 pt 1):324-331.

Nygaard I, Thom DH, Calhoun E. Urinary incontinence in women. In: Litwin M, Saigal C, eds. *Urologic Diseases in America.* Washington, D.C.: U.S. Government Publishing Office; 2004:71-103.

Thom DH, Nygaard IE, Calhoun EA. Urologic diseases in America project: urinary incontinence in women—national trends in hospitalizations, office visits, treatment and economic impact. *J Urol.* 2005;173:1295-1301.

Preoperative Evaluation of Patients with Urinary Incontinence and Selection of Appropriate Surgical Procedures for Stress Incontinence

2

W. Stuart Reynolds, M.D.
Mickey Karram, M.D.
Roger Dmochowski, M.D.

Preoperative Evaluation

The evaluation of a patient with urinary incontinence (UI) is focused on characterizing the incontinence, identifying any concomitant or contributory factors, and determining the patient's treatment goals and preferences to direct initial treatment decision making and counseling. Essential elements in the initial assessment include a focused medical history and physical examination and basic clinical testing. Additional elements may be necessary if UI is poorly characterized or additional findings suggest a more complicated situation (**Video 2-1**).

History

Evaluation of patients with UI begins with a thorough history and review of the medical record. Elements of the history should be directed toward determining the type of UI (stress urinary incontinence [SUI], urge urinary incontinence [UUI], or mixed incontinence [MUI]) and assessing the duration, frequency, and severity of incontinence episodes; impact of symptoms on lifestyle; and patient expectations of treatment. In addition, the patient should be questioned regarding the presence of other lower urinary tract symptoms and concomitant bowel and pelvic conditions, which may be contributory. Prior treatments for UI, if any, should be reviewed in detail (**Videos 2-2** and **2-3**). Finally, obstetric, surgical, bowel, and medication histories should be reviewed with the patient to identify any complicating factors or comorbidity that may have an impact on treatment options. Symptoms of other pelvic floor disorders, such as pelvic organ prolapse (POP), defecatory dysfunction, pelvic pain, and sexual dysfunction, should also be sought.

Questionnaires and Symptom Measurement Tools

Several tools are available for further assessment and quantification of symptoms, severity, and health-related quality of life (QOL) issues. A simple frequency volume chart or bladder diary is generally recommended to document the frequency and volumes of voiding, incontinence episodes, and use of incontinence pads. Patient-reported symptom and QOL questionnaires may be used to assess the patient's perspective regarding symptoms and effects on QOL. Although many questionnaires are available, the use of high-quality, robustly validated tools is recommended by most professional societies. Commonly used instruments are presented in the Appendix, including Urogenital Distress Inventory-6 (UDI-6), Incontinence Impact Questionnaire-7 (IIQ-7), International Consultation on Incontinence Modular Questionnaire–Short Form (ICIQ-SF), Incontinence Quality of Life Instrument (I-QOL), and American Urological Association Symptom Index (Abrams et al., 2010).

Physical Examination

As part of the initial assessment, a thorough physical examination should be performed with special attention paid to the lower abdomen and pelvis. Components of overall health status include assessment of mental status, obesity (body mass index), and physical dexterity and mobility. Abdominal examination should assess for masses, bladder distention, and relevant surgical scars. Genitourinary examination should include an overall assessment of genital anatomy and neurologic function. The presence of urine leakage from the urethral meatus should be confirmed, if possible, in patients describing SUI symptoms; extraurethral leakage (fistula formation) should always be considered in patients who have had previous surgery or radiation. The vagina should be inspected to assess estrogen status, for concomitant POP, and, if relevant, for the presence of any foreign body or material (**Videos 2-4** and **2-5**).

Cough Test

Provocative testing for SUI can confirm the presence of the sign of SUI and is usually done with a cough or provocative stress test. The cough stress test can be performed with the bladder empty or filled and with the patient supine or standing. For the test, the patient is asked to cough vigorously several times while the examiner observes for urine loss from the meatus. Any leakage of urine with provocation is considered a positive test. Ideally, the bladder is filled up to 300 mL or to a sense of fullness; however, the test can also be performed with an empty bladder. In the supine empty stress test, the patient voids immediately before examination in the lithotomy position and coughs or strains (Valsalva maneuver) while the examiner inspects the urethral meatus. In either the full or the empty test, if leakage does not occur in the supine lithotomy position, the patient repeats the maneuvers in the standing position. Some studies have correlated a positive empty supine stress test with objective urodynamics testing indicative of intrinsic sphincter deficiency (**Videos 2-3** and **2-6**).

Hypermobility

Some debate surrounds the role of urethral hypermobility or lack thereof in the assessment of SUI. Urethral hypermobility refers to the degree of rotation and descent of the urethra away from its retropubic position with increased abdominal pressure and is considered a sign of loss of urethral support. When urine leakage occurs without urethral hypermobility, primary urethral sphincter weakness (i.e., intrinsic sphincter deficiency) is suspected.

The cotton-tipped swab (Q-tip) test was designed to quantify the degree of hypermobility by measuring the angle of deflection from horizontal of the swab inserted into the urethra during cough or Valsalva maneuver. To perform the test, a swab is inserted per the urethra to the level of the urethrovesical junction, and the angle of the swab compared with horizontal is assessed. Next, the patient coughs or strains, and the change in the angle of the swab is noted. An excursion of 30 degrees or more is a positive test for hypermobility. Although this test is not a diagnostic test, it is an objective measure for quantifying bladder neck mobility during excursion (**Video 2-7** and Figure 2-1).

Pelvic Organ Prolapse

The degree of POP should be described using common grading and staging methods. The two most common methods include the POP quantification and Baden-Walker systems. Both methods attempt to standardize the description and

Q-tip test

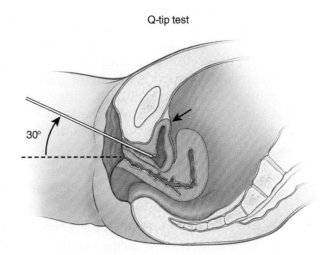

Figure 2-1 Cotton-tipped swab (Q-tip) test. As the patient bears down, the cotton swab moves, and the angle of deflection can be measured *(arrow)*. In this example, it is 30 degrees, indicating urethral hypermobility. A measurement of 30 degrees or more from baseline (which in this case is 0 degrees from the horizontal) is considered to signify hypermobility. The *curved arrow* indicates the deflection or movement of the cotton swab with abdominal straining.

(From Nitti VW, ed. Vaginal Surgery for the Urologist. *Philadelphia: Saunders; 2012. Female Pelvic Surgery Video Atlas Series.)*

degree of pelvic organ descent, using the hymen as a fixed point of reference. Staging by the POP quantification system is assigned according to the most severe portion of the prolapse: stage 0, no prolapse is demonstrated; stage I, the most distal portion of the prolapse is greater than 1 cm above the level of the hymen; stage II, the most distal portion of the prolapse is less than 1 cm below the hymen; stage III, the most distal portion of the prolapse is greater than 1 cm below the plane of the hymen; stage IV, there is complete eversion of the total length of the lower genital tract. For a more detailed description of these prolapse staging methods, refer to the book entitled *Surgical Management of Pelvic Organ Prolapse*, edited by Karram and Maher, in the Pelvic Surgery Video Atlas Series (2012).

Clinical Testing

Basic clinical testing should be performed to confirm the symptoms and findings of the history and physical examination and to rule out any complicating factors or conditions that may have an impact on treatment decision making.

Urinalysis

In all patients with urinary symptoms, including incontinence, urinalysis to assess for the presence of infection or blood should be considered because infection may be a readily treatable cause of symptoms, and blood may suggest complicated etiologies warranting further evaluation. Methods include dipstick testing, microscopic examination of the urinary sediment, and culture, if indicated.

Post-Void Volume Measure

Measurement of post-void residual bladder volume is recommended to assess bladder emptying and urine retention, as signs for underlying bladder function abnormalities. Common methods include ultrasound and bladder catheterization.

Pad Testing

To quantify the amount of urine loss, pad testing or weighing, in which the patient collects and submits incontinence pads worn for a prescribed interval to be weighed, can be performed, although this is considered to be an optional test in most clinical settings. It is very helpful when assessing and comparing the results of the treatment of different types of incontinence in different centers. The International Continence Society recommends a test spanning a 1-hour period during which a series of standardized activities are carried out. A typical test schedule includes the following:

1. Test is started without the subject voiding.
2. A preweighed collecting device is put on when the 1-hour test period begins.
3. The subject drinks 500 mL of sodium-free liquid within a short period (maximum 15 minutes), and then sits or rests.
4. At 30 minutes, the subject walks, including stair climbing equivalent to one flight up and down.
5. During the remaining 30 minutes, the subject performs the following activities:
   a. Standing up from sitting, 10 times
   b. Coughing vigorously, 10 times

c. Running in place for 1 minute

d. Bending to pick up small objects from floor, 5 times

e. Washing hands in running water for 1 minute

6. At the end of the 1-hour test, the collecting device is removed and weighed.

7. If the test is regarded as representative, the subject voids, and the volume is recorded.

8. Otherwise the test is repeated preferably without voiding.

Office Evaluation of Bladder Filling: "Eyeball" Cystometry

An office evaluation of UI should involve some assessment of voiding, detrusor function during filling, and assessment of urethral competency. This evaluation can be performed using a 50-mL syringe without its piston or bulb, a bottle of water, and a red rubber catheter. The examination is best initiated with the patient's bladder comfortably full. The patient is allowed to void as normally as possible in private. The time to void and the amount of urine voided are recorded. The patient returns to the examination room, and the volume of residual urine is noted by transurethral catheterization (a sterile urine sample can be obtained for analysis at this time). The patient is asked to sit up, and the bladder is filled by gravity by pouring 50-mL aliquots of sterile water into the syringe (Figure 2-2). The patient's first bladder sensation and maximum bladder capacity are noted. The water level in the syringe should be closely observed during filling because any rise in the column of water can be

Figure 2-2 "Eyeball" cystometry. Office evaluation of bladder filling function. With the patient in a sitting or standing position with a catheter in the bladder, the bladder is filled by gravity by pouring sterile water into the syringe.

(From Walters MD, Karram MM, eds. Urogynecology and Reconstructive Pelvic Surgery, *ed 3. Philadelphia: Mosby; 2007.)*

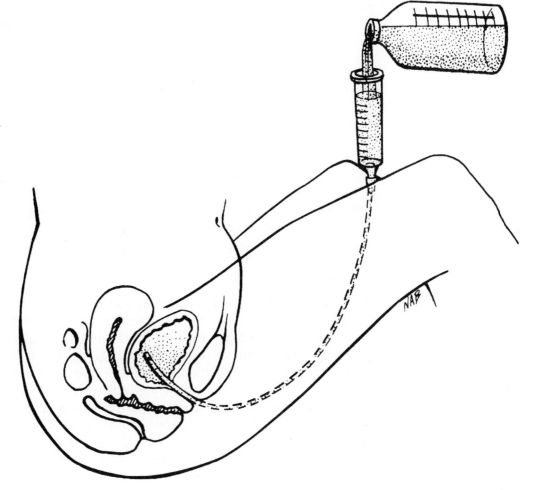

secondary to a detrusor contraction. Unintended increases in intraabdominal pressure by the patient should be avoided. The catheter is removed, and the patient is asked to cough in a standing position. Loss of small amounts of urine in spurts simultaneous with coughs strongly suggests a diagnosis of urodynamic SUI, whereas leaking a few seconds after coughing or no urine loss with provocation indicates that other causes of incontinence, especially detrusor overactivity, may be the cause of incontinence.

This simple filling "eyeball" study almost always reproduces the sign of stress incontinence in women who have urodynamic SUI. It also provides information on voiding efficiency and function and bladder capacity and sensation (**Video 2-6**).

Advanced Testing

Advanced testing or invasive diagnostic procedures should be considered when basic assessment fails to characterize the incontinence accurately or additional, complicating factors are identified that might determine appropriate direction for care.

Urodynamics

Multichannel urodynamics testing is warranted in cases where results may change management, such as before most invasive treatments, and in cases of complicated UI, including after prior treatment failure; when neurogenic lower urinary tract dysfunction is present; and when incontinence is associated with additional lower urinary tract symptoms, such as advanced prolapse, hematuria, pain, recurrent urinary tract infections, or a history of radical pelvic surgery or radiation therapy. Urodynamics testing is generally performed in a dedicated laboratory with specially trained personnel. The mainstay of urodynamics involves measuring the pressure-volume relationship (cystometry) during bladder filling and emptying.

The goals of any urodynamics evaluation are as follows:

1. Reproduce symptoms and correlate symptoms with urodynamic findings.
2. Assess bladder sensation.
3. Attempt to detect detrusor overactivity.
4. Assess urethral competence during filling and with provocation.
5. Ensure appropriate synergy between detrusor muscle and outlet.
6. Determine detrusor function during voiding.
7. Assess outlet function during voiding.
8. Measure residual urine.

See **Video 2-8** for a discussion of specific urodynamics tests.

During the urodynamics procedure, intravesical and intraabdominal pressures are simultaneously measured via multichannel catheters inserted into the urethra and vagina or rectum during bladder filling (filling cystometry) and emptying (pressure-flow measurements). Subtraction of abdominal pressure from vesical pressure results in true detrusor pressure. After the catheters are placed under sterile technique, the patient is typically seated, and the bladder is filled with saline at a continuous rate (Figure 2-3). During cystometry, both the patient and the health care provider give information to elicit the desired measurements and findings, which typically include sensation, bladder capacity, resting pressure and compliance, and the presence of uninhibited bladder

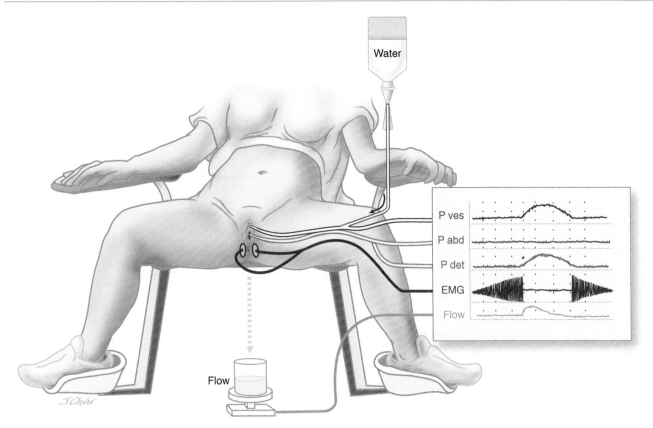

Figure 2-3 Setup for urodynamics testing. The patient is typically seated on the urodynamics chair after the catheters have been placed. Abdominal and vesical pressures are measured by catheters in the bladder and vagina or rectum. The machine automatically calculates true detrusor pressure *(P det)* by subtracting intraabdominal pressure *(P abd)* from intravesical pressure *(P ves)*. Electromyography *(EMG)* activity using surface electrodes and urinary flow are also measured.

contractions. Provocative maneuvers (cough test and Valsalva maneuver) can be incorporated to assess for stress incontinence, including determination of leak point pressure measurements. Alternatively, urethral pressure profilometry can be performed with a specialized urethral catheter to assess for urethral length and closure pressures.

Once capacity is reached, the patient voids into a calibrated uroflowmeter to measure flow rates (peak or maximum and average) and voided volume. By leaving the bladder catheter in place during voiding, concomitant detrusor pressures (maximum and pressure at maximum flow) can also be measured as part of pressure-flow studies. For either method, post-void residual urine volume is determined.

Additional components of urodynamics include urinary sphincter electromyography (EMG) and fluoroscopy (videourodynamics). EMG allows simultaneous measurement of urethral sphincter function, which is particularly important in the setting of neurologic conditions to document the presence of detrusor-sphincter dyssynergia. The addition of fluoroscopy allows for lower urinary tract imaging during filling and voiding to identify anatomic abnormalities, including vesicoureteral reflux, bladder neck function, diverticula, or fistula. Figure 2-4 illustrates examples of storage and micturition reflexes in a neurologically intact patient.

Cystoscopy

Cystourethroscopy is warranted when initial assessment identifies abnormalities of the urinary system or urine sediment for which direct visualization of the lower urinary tract is indicated, such as hematuria, or when symptoms

Typical Storage Reflex

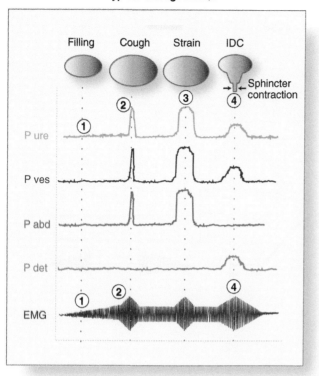

Typical Micturition Reflex

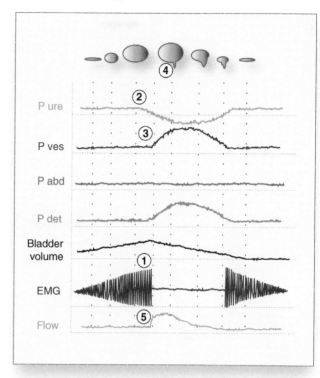

A

B

Figure 2-4 A, Typical storage reflex in a neurologically intact woman; note increased electromyography *(EMG)* activity during filling, provocation, and an uninhibited detrusor contraction. This indicates an intact synergist pelvic floor response. **B,** Typical micturition reflex in a neurologically intact woman. Note complete loss of EMG activity simultaneous with an increase in detrusor pressure at initiation of voiding. *IDC,* Involuntary detrusor contraction; *P abd,* intraabdominal pressure; *P det,* detrusor pressure; *P ure,* urethral pressure; *P ves,* intravesical pressure.

suggest an intravesical lesion, including mass, foreign body, or fistula. Visual inspection of urethra and bladder can identify urethral stricture and sources of bladder outlet obstruction, bladder mucosal tumors, foreign bodies involving the lower urinary tract, fistula, and diverticula.

Imaging

Radiologic testing is not recommended for cases of uncomplicated UI; however, several modalities are useful in complicated cases of pelvic floor dysfunction, including after failed surgery and in cases in which upper urinary tract or renal pathology may be present. Imaging may be performed with renal and pelvic ultrasonography; cystourethrography, including during urodynamics (videourodynamics); computed tomography (CT); and pelvic magnetic resonance imaging (MRI).

Perioperative Considerations

Antibiotic Prophylaxis

More recent guidelines on antimicrobial prophylaxis to prevent surgical site infections and urinary tract infections recommend periprocedural systemic administration of antibiotics for most procedures performed for surgical treatment of UI. All urinary tract procedures are considered clean-contaminated, suggesting that bacteria may be present at the site of the procedure at the time of incision, despite sterile preparation of the surgical site. With few exceptions, antimicrobial prophylaxis is unnecessary after wound closure or on termination of endoscopic procedures and should not extend beyond 24 hours after a procedure. Possible exceptions include the placement of prosthetic material; the presence of an existing infection; and the manipulation of an indwelling tube, such as an indwelling bladder (Foley) catheter or ureteral stent. Common antimicrobial regimens include parenteral first-generation or second-generation cephalosporins, fluoroquinolones, or an aminoglycoside plus metronidazole or clindamycin. Antibiotics should be administered within 1 hour of incision.

Deep Vein Thrombosis Prevention

Although risks for developing deep vein thrombosis and pulmonary embolism often depend on patient-specific risk factors, thrombosis prophylaxis during antiincontinence and pelvic reconstructive surgery has been shown to decrease the occurrence. The nature of the procedure also plays a role because the risks of deep vein thrombosis and pulmonary embolism are generally low for endoscopic procedures (i.e., cystourethroscopy and urethral bulking) and suburethral slings (i.e., synthetic midurethral sling [MUS]). High-risk surgeries include anterior and posterior vaginal wall repairs, uterosacral vault suspension, sacrospinous ligament fixation, paravaginal repair, and abdominal sacrocolpopexy. For moderate-risk to high-risk patients (i.e., patients >40 years old with additional risk factors or all patients >60 years old), the use of intermittent pneumatic compression, low-dose unfractionated heparin, or low-molecular-weight heparin may be considered separately (moderate-risk patients) or in combination (high-risk patients).

Case 1: Index Stress Urinary Incontinence Patient

Scenario

The patient is a 45-year-old, healthy woman who reports progressive worsening of urinary leakage with exercise and vigorous coughing over the past 8 months. Incontinent episodes occur weekly with small amounts of urine loss, not in association with urgency or frequency. She has had three prior vaginal deliveries but no pelvic surgeries and takes no medications. Her body size is ideal, and the genitourinary examination is normal with the exception of urine leakage on vigorous cough with a subjectively full bladder. There is obvious mobility of the urethra. She is interested in definitive treatment.

Evaluation

This is the index patient with SUI. With complaints consistent with demonstrable incontinence on examination and no apparent complicating factors, a limited evaluation is warranted for this patient. A urinalysis and post-void residual measurement for screening purposes and an "eyeball" filling study to objectify the sign of stress incontinence should be considered. In our opinion, treatment could proceed without more involved testing.

Treatment Options

A range of treatment options would be applicable in this scenario. Factors to consider and discuss with the patient include morbidity of any proposed procedure, longevity and duration of results, and potential risks for adverse events. Urethral bulking (see Chapter 9) could be considered, particularly if minimal invasiveness is desired, although durability of results would be an issue in a young, healthy, active woman. Any suburethral sling whether synthetic or biologic would be an option, including a biologic pubovaginal sling (see Chapter 5), retropubic (see Chapter 6) or transobturator (see Chapter 7) synthetic MUS, or single-incision minisling (see Chapter 8). A retropubic operation (see Chapter 4), although feasible, would likely incur higher morbidity than necessary with the availability of less morbid options. Available long-term outcome data for these various procedures and patient preference regarding degree of morbidity and risk profile of the possible options should drive decision making in this instance. We would most likely elect to perform a transobturator or retropubic synthetic sling on such an index SUI patient.

Case 2: Patient with Mixed Urinary Incontinence

Scenario

A 58-year-old woman complains of urine leakage both with activity and exercise and with urgency. She is most bothered by the stress incontinence because this happens more frequently (weekly); urgency and urge incontinence occur less often. She has never been treated surgically, but she takes an anticholinergic medication presently with some benefit. Her medical history is significant for two vaginal deliveries but otherwise noncontributory. On genitourinary examination, she demonstrates urethral hypermobility, urinary leakage with cough, and mild asymptomatic (stage 1) anterior prolapse; there are no other abnormalities. She is interested in definitive treatment.

Evaluation

Urinalysis with microscopy and post-void urine residual measurement should be performed in this patient to screen for other abnormalities that may be contributory to bladder overactivity. Urodynamics and cystoscopy should also be considered for this patient before performing any invasive treatment.

On urodynamics testing, this patient was found to have a normal-capacity bladder with uninhibited detrusor contractions and stress incontinence on provocative testing during filling. Voiding-pressure assessment was normal with complete bladder emptying. Cystoscopy demonstrated no abnormality.

Treatment Options

Because SUI is more bothersome than UUI in this patient, offering a surgical intervention is a reasonable approach. Several treatment options can be considered for this patient with classic MUI, as follows: MUS, including retropubic (see Chapter 6), transobturator (see Chapter 7), or single-incision minisling (see Chapter 8); pubovaginal sling (see Chapter 5); a retropubic suspension (see Chapter 4); and urethral bulking (see Chapter 9). In counseling the patient regarding treatment options, the surgeon should consider the effects of various procedures on urinary urgency, including resolution, worsening, or no change in symptoms. In addition, results (cure or improvement in overall incontinence) may not be as good as for a patient without the urgency component, and this should be discussed and the patient should understand that there might be a worsening of her urge symptoms. As a general rule, 50% of women with MUI have resolution of urge symptoms, 25% have no change, and 25% have worsening of their symptoms after MUS.

Case 3: Recurrent Stress Urinary Incontinence

Scenario

A 53-year-old woman reports recurrence of UI after having undergone a transobturator MUS 4 years previously. Although initially continent after surgery, she has noted worsening incontinence for the past 12 months, both in frequency of episodes and in amount of urine leakage. Incontinence episodes typically occur with physical activity or coughing (SUI), and she wears a daily pad. She denies urgency or UUI as well as other symptoms, such as hesitancy, dysuria, incomplete emptying, or hematuria. She is otherwise healthy with no recent changes to her health or additional procedures since the initial MUS. On genitourinary examination, her vagina is healthy-appearing without foreign body exposure or fistula; grade 1 asymptomatic anterior POP is present, but no urine leakage is seen despite cough testing and the presence of urethral hypermobility with cough and straining. Urinalysis is normal, and post-void residual by ultrasound is 30 mL.

Evaluation

Urodynamics is generally recommended in this scenario of prior surgical treatment. Also, in this case without demonstrable SUI on examination, urodynamics may help provide objective evidence for SUI. Although the patient's complaints do not suggest voiding dysfunction or bladder overactivity, urodynamics in the postoperative setting would be an effective way to screen for obstructive voiding or uninhibited detrusor contractions. Cystoscopy is also recommended to evaluate for possible sling material exposure or extrusion into the lower urinary tract and other potential causes of incontinence, such as urethral diverticulum. In this scenario, urodynamics confirmed SUI without associated voiding abnormalities, and cystoscopy was normal.

Treatment Options

In the setting of uncomplicated recurrence of SUI, several options are available, including urethral bulking (see Chapter 9), repeat MUS (see Chapters 6-8), or pubovaginal sling (see Chapter 5). Selecting a particular intervention is determined in part by the patient's preferences and willingness to undergo additional invasive treatment. The degree of urethral hypermobility versus primary urethral sphincter weakness (intrinsic sphincter deficiency) may also determine treatment options. In this scenario, the patient has recurrent SUI with hypermobility, suggesting a worsening of urethral support. Because she had failed a previous transobturator MUS, we would most likely proceed with a retropubic MUS or an autologous pubovaginal sling placed underneath the bladder neck. If no hypermobility were present, suggesting intrinsic sphincter deficiency, urethral bulking would be an option. Experts debate whether removal of the existing sling or urethrolysis should be performed before or in conjunction with an additional antiincontinence procedure.

Figures 2-5 and 2-6 are urodynamics tracings demonstrating uninhibited bladder contractions and urodynamic SUI.

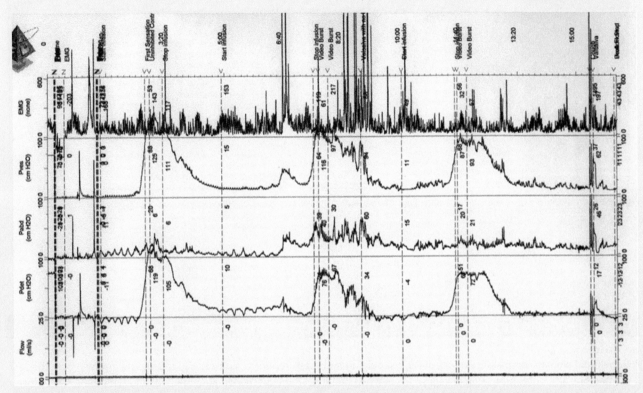

Figure 2-5 Urodynamics tracing. During filling cystometry, several uninhibited detrusor contractions occur, with amplitudes of 72 to 119 cm H_2O, consistent with detrusor overactivity.

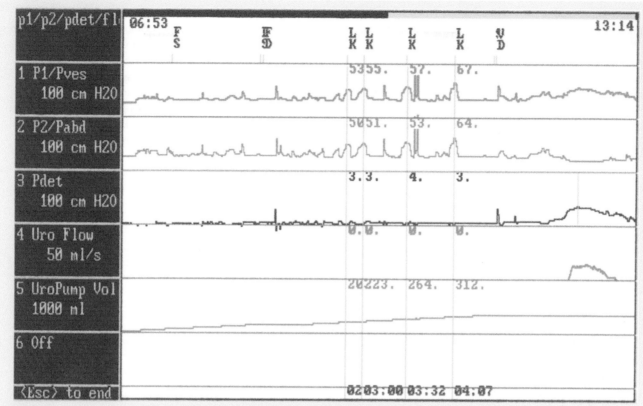

Figure 2-6 Urodynamic tracing. SUI is present with cough and Valsalva maneuver testing, with abdominal leak point pressures of 50 to 64 cm H$_2$O.

Case 4: Pelvic Organ Prolapse and Occult Stress Urinary Incontinence

Scenario

A 62-year-old woman complains primarily of vaginal bulging and pressure, which has been progressively worsening over the past 8 months. She also notes protrusion of vaginal tissue when bathing. When questioned about her voiding symptoms, she states that she has had UI mostly related to activity (SUI) in the past, but this has improved over the last year or so. Now she does not leak but has hesitancy, intermittency, and the feeling of incomplete emptying after voiding. She has a history of vaginal delivery (one) and cesarean sections (two) and underwent a vaginal hysterectomy for uterine fibroids 15 years ago. She otherwise is well and has had no other surgeries or medical conditions. On examination, she is overweight (body mass index = 29). She has no other abnormal findings on abdominal examination. On genitourinary examination, she has stage 3 anterior and apical prolapse with urethral hypermobility but no leakage with cough testing. Urinalysis is normal, and post-void residual by ultrasound is 140 mL.

Evaluation

In the setting of advanced POP, urodynamics testing is recommended to assess for voiding dysfunction. In this scenario, the patient is complaining of symptoms suggestive of obstructive voiding with a remote history of SUI. Urodynamics should be able to quantify the degree of bladder and voiding dysfunction. In addition, if not performed during physical examination, POP reduction and provocative testing during urodynamics should be performed to identify the presence of occult SUI. Additional testing with fluoroscopy during urodynamics (videourodynamics) or renal ultrasonography should be considered to evaluate for upper urinary tract changes in the setting of presumed urinary obstruction.

A representative urodynamics tracing is presented in Figure 2-7. Initially, on filling cystometry, significant POP and vesicoureteral reflux were noted, while on voiding pressure studies, obstruction and incomplete emptying were present. After POP reduction, SUI was present with provocative testing, and normal, low-pressure voiding ensued. Cystourethroscopy was normal.

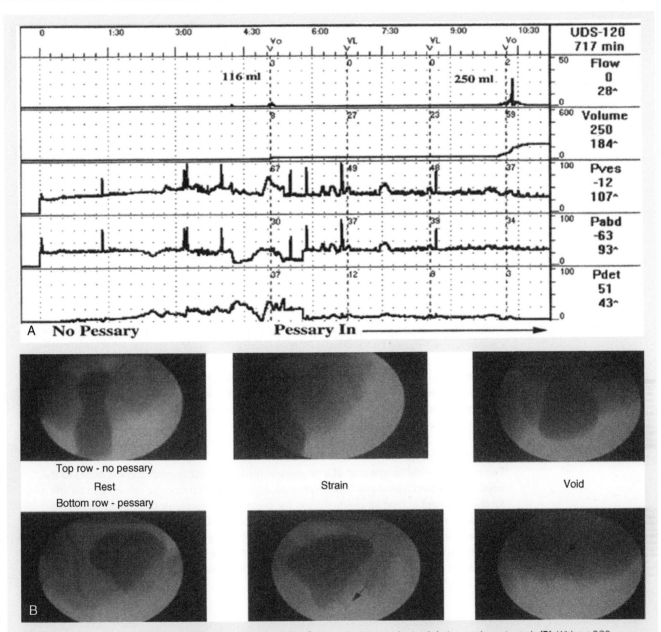

Figure 2-7 Urodynamic tracing **(A)** and pre/post pessary placement fluoroscopic images obtained during urodynamic study **(B).** Without POP reduction, no leakage is seen with cough testing, and obstructed voiding (high detrusor pressure and low flow) is present. When a pessary is inserted to reduce POP, SUI is evident, and low-pressure voiding is achieved.

Treatment Options

Treatment of this patient's POP is warranted and could be performed with many surgical options, which are beyond the focus of this discussion. A concurrent antiincontinence procedure should be performed in conjunction with the repair of POP, given the finding of occult SUI. Multiple options are reasonable for this patient, including a retropubic suspension (see Chapter 4) or a pubovaginal (see Chapter 5) or midurethral (see Chapters 6-8) sling. Choice of a particular procedure may be determined by the approach to POP repair and patient and surgeon preferences.

Case 5: Neurogenic Bladder

Scenario

A 46-year-old paraplegic woman who sustained a spinal cord injury at level T-12 4 years ago performs self-intermittent catheterization every 6 hours but complains of worsening incontinence between catheterizations. She currently takes a daily oral anticholinergic medication for uninhibited bladder contractions and has been on her current treatment regimen for 2 years. She also complains of some leakage with activity, specifically when transferring into and out of her wheelchair. She has had several urinary tract infections in the past 6 months that have been treated with oral antibiotic therapy. She has had no prior pelvic surgeries or therapies for UI. On examination, she has normal-appearing genitalia but has incontinence with cough and Valsalva maneuver associated with urethral hypermobility.

Evaluation

In the setting of a neurologic condition affecting the lower urinary tract (i.e., neurogenic bladder), urodynamics evaluation is recommended to assess for changes in bladder function, particularly if symptoms change, as in this patient. The addition of fluoroscopy (videourodynamics) can help to identify vesicoureteral reflux and potential damage to the upper urinary tract and kidney function. Upper tract imaging (renal ultrasound) should also be considered to assess for hydronephrosis and changes to the kidney (e.g., parenchymal loss or cortical thinning). Measurement of serum creatinine levels should be considered if upper urinary tract or renal abnormalities are noted. Urodynamics testing for this patient is shown in Figure 2-8. Important findings include a low maximum bladder capacity (150 mL), elevated resting bladder pressure (30 to 45 cm H_2O), uninhibited bladder contractions associated with urine leakage, and lack of coordination between bladder contraction and sphincter relaxation (detrusor-sphincter dyssynergia). The fluoroscopic component reveals mild ureteral reflux and hydronephrosis.

Treatment Options

This patient has had progression of a neurogenic bladder condition, with some changes to the upper urinary tract (reflux and hydronephrosis). Although anticholinergic therapy can be effective for the treatment of bladder overactivity in the presence of neurologic conditions, additional therapies are warranted in this case to improve bladder capacity, decrease resting bladder pressures, and decrease incontinence episodes. A trial of high-dose botulinum toxin injection to the bladder can be considered; however, many patients ultimately require bladder augmentation (see Chapter 10). SUI may also be present, requiring closure of the bladder outlet with a compressive pubovaginal sling (see Chapter 5).

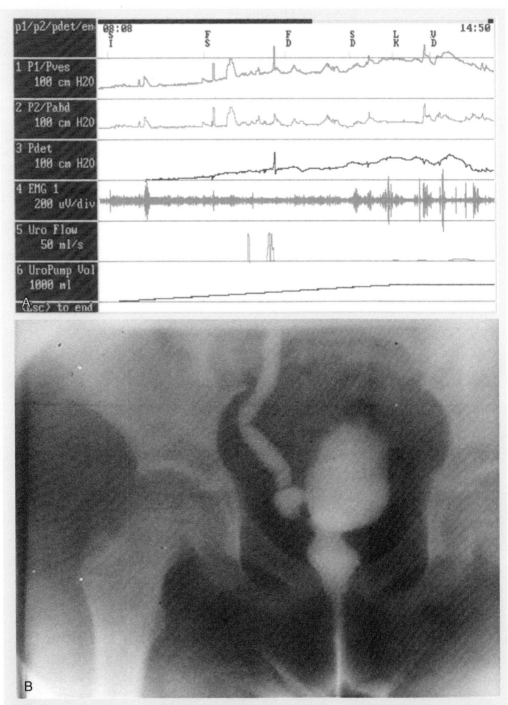

Figure 2-8 A, Urodynamics tracing. On filling cystometry, elevated detrusor pressures are present along with low capacity and spontaneous leakage near capacity, consistent with findings of a neurogenic bladder. **B,** On fluoroscopy images, unilateral vesicoureteral reflux is visible on the patient's right.

Suggested Readings

Abrams P, Andersson KE, Birder L, et al. Fourth International Consultation on Incontinence Recommendations of the International Scientific Committee: evaluation and treatment of urinary incontinence, pelvic organ prolapse, and fecal incontinence. *Neurourol Urodyn*. 2010;29:213-240.

Dmochowski RR, Blaivas JM, Gormley EA, et al. Update of AUA guideline on the surgical management of female stress urinary incontinence. *J Urol*. 2010;183:1906-1914.

Forrest JB, Clemens JQ, Finamore P, et al. AUA Best Practice Statement for the prevention of deep vein thrombosis in patients undergoing urologic surgery. *J Urol*. 2009;181:1170-1177.

Ghoniem G, Stanford E, Kenton K, et al. Evaluation and outcome measures in the treatment of female urinary stress incontinence: International Urogynecological Association (IUGA) guidelines for research and clinical practice. *Int Urogynecol J Pelvic Floor Dysfunct*. 2008;19:5-33.

Haylen BT, De Ridder D, Freeman RM, et al. An International Urogynecological Association (IUGA)/International Continence Society (ICS) joint report on the terminology for female pelvic floor dysfunction. *Neurourol Urodyn*. 2010;29:4-20.

Karram M, Maher CF. *Surgical Management of Pelvic Organ Prolapse: Female Pelvic Surgery Video Atlas Series*. Philadelphia: Saunders; 2013.

Wolf JS, Bennett CJ, Dmochowski RR, et al. Best practice policy statement on urologic surgery antimicrobial prophylaxis. *J Urol*. 2008;179:1379-1390.

Surgical Anatomy of the Anterior Vaginal Wall, Retropubic Space, and Inner Groin

Mickey Karram, M.D.

Videos

3-1 Anatomy of the Anterior Vaginal Wall
3-2 Anatomy of the Lower Urinary Tract
3-3 Anatomy of Retropubic Space (Cadaveric Dissection)
3-4 Anatomy of Retropubic Space (Live Surgical Demonstration)

3-5 Anatomy Relevant to Retropubic Midurethral Slings
3-6 Anatomy Relevant to Transobturator Midurethral Slings

Introduction

A surgeon performing the various procedures for urinary incontinence that are discussed in this book should be very familiar with the anatomy and dissection planes required to perform these procedures in a safe and efficient fashion. This chapter will review the anatomy of the anterior vaginal wall, the lower urinary tract, the retropubic space, and the inner groin.

Anatomy of Anterior Vaginal Wall

When performing suburethral sling procedures for stress urinary incontinence, fully appreciating the relationship between the anterior vaginal wall and the posterior urethra and bladder becomes very important in regard to establishing appropriate planes of dissection (**Video 3-1**). Synthetic midurethral slings have become very popular for the correction of stress incontinence. These slings are placed in the distal to mid urethra; this dissection plane is a completely different dissection plane than the plane of dissection under the proximal urethra and bladder neck. The distal portion of the anterior vaginal wall is just superior to the perineal membrane and is fused with the posterior wall of the urethra. An appropriate dissection plane requires sharp dissection to elucidate fully the plane in which the sling is placed (see **Video 3-1**). As the dissection extends toward the bladder neck, there is a much clearer plane of dissection between the proximal urethra and the anterior vaginal wall and subsequently between the vaginal wall and the wall of the bladder. The vagina lies anteriorly adjacent to and supports the bladder base, from which it is separated by the vesicovaginal adventitia (endopelvic fascia). The urethra is fused with the anterior vagina, with no distinct adventitial layer separating them. The terminal portions of the ureters cross the lateral fornices of the vagina on their way to the bladder base (Figure 3-1). Dissection in the middle third of the anterior vaginal wall can be either superficial to the fibromuscular layer of the vagina, within the fibromuscular layer of the vagina, or deeper in the true vesicovaginal space. The dissection of the deeper vesicovaginal space separates the vaginal wall from the overlying trigone. In the authors' opinion, the best dissection plan when performing a traditional anterior colporrhaphy is to be within the fibromuscular layer of the vagina because this plane is the least vascular and allows appropriate plication without significant distortion of the trigone or irritation of the visceral innervation of the bladder. If mesh

Figure 3-1 The rectum and the posterior wall of the vagina have been excised. The relationship of the ureters and bladder base to the anterior and anterolateral vagina is illustrated. Urinary tract structures are pink. If the picture is inverted, the relationship of the urethra and the vestibule to the anterior vagina can be better understood.

(From Baggish MS, Karram MM, eds. Atlas of Pelvic Anatomy and Gynecologic Surgery, *ed 3. St. Louis: Saunders; 2011.)*

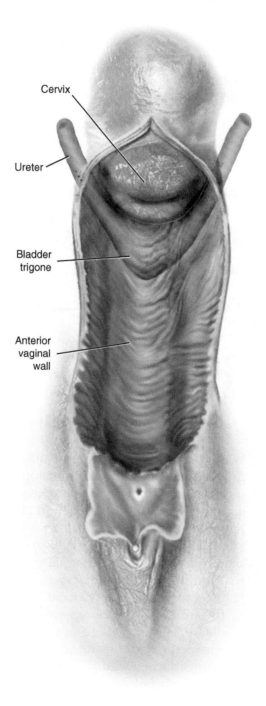

Cervix

Ureter

Bladder trigone

Anterior vaginal wall

augmentation is to be used, some surgeons believe that placing the mesh in the deeper vesicovaginal space decreases the chance for subsequent vaginal mesh erosion.

Anatomy of the Lower Urinary Tract

Traditionally, support of the urethra and bladder neck was thought to be provided by the interaction of the pubourethral ligaments, the perineal membrane, and the muscles of the pelvic floor. Milley and Nichols (1971) found bilaterally symmetric anterior, posterior, and intermediate pubourethral ligaments and stated that the anterior and posterior ligaments were formed by inferior and superior fascial layers of the perineal membrane. An anatomic defect of the pubourethral ligaments has been cited as a contributing factor to stress urinary incontinence and is thought to be in part (based on the integral theory of Ulmsten and Petros, 1995) why synthetic midurethral slings surgically correct stress incontinence. Studies by DeLancey (1986, 1988, 1989) showed that rather than being suspended ventrally by ligamentous structures, the proximal urethra and bladder base are supported in a slinglike fashion by the anterior vaginal wall, which is attached bilaterally to the levator ani muscles, at the arcus tendineus fasciae pelvis. These attachments extend caudally and blend with the superior fibers of the perineal membrane. The tissues described as pubourethral ligaments are made up of the perineal membrane and the most caudal portion of the arcus tendineus fasciae pelvis, which fix the distal urethra beneath the pubic bone. Figure 3-2 illustrates the anatomic structures that contribute to urethral support and closure. The attachment of the anterior vaginal wall at the arcus tendineus fasciae pelvis may contribute to urethral closure by providing a stable base onto which the urethra is compressed with increases in intraabdominal pressure. These attachments are also responsible for the posterior movement of the vesical neck seen at the onset of micturition and for the elevation noted when the patient is instructed to perform a Kegel exercise or interrupt her urinary stream. Defects in these attachments result in urethral hypermobility and anterior vaginal wall prolapse.

The female urethra is about 4 cm long and averages 6 mm in diameter. Its lumen is slightly curved as it passes from the retropubic space, perforates the perineal membrane, and ends with its external orifice in the vestibule directly above the vaginal opening. Throughout its length, the urethra is embedded in the adventitia of the anterior vagina. The epithelium of the urethra is continuous externally with the epithelium of the vulva and internally with the epithelium of the bladder. Most of the epithelium is stratified squamous but becomes transitional near the bladder. The entire urethra is composed of smooth muscle, which is primarily oblique and longitudinal muscle fibers. This smooth muscle and the detrusor muscle in the bladder base form the intrinsic urethral sphincter mechanism. The striated urethral and periurethral muscles form the extrinsic urethral sphincter mechanism. The inner portion of this sphincter is made up of a striated band of muscle that surrounds the proximal two thirds of the urethra and the compressor urethral and urethrovaginal sphincter, which consists of two straplike bands of striated muscle that arch over the ventral surface of the distal one third of the urethra (see Figure 3-2). Oelrich (1983) termed these three muscles the striated urogenital sphincter. These muscles contribute (along with the levator ani) to voluntary interruption of urine and to urethral closure with increases in abdominal pressure via a reflex muscle contraction.

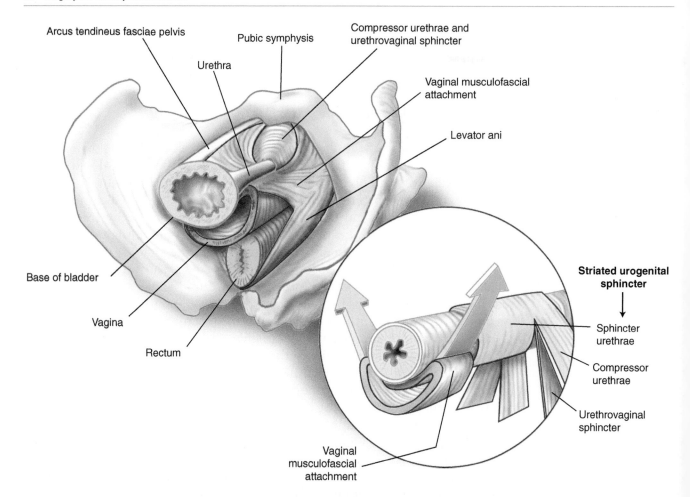

Arcus tendineus fasciae pelvis

Pubic symphysis

Compressor urethrae and
urethrovaginal sphincter

Urethra

Vaginal musculofascial
attachment

Levator ani

Base of bladder

Vagina

Rectum

**Striated urogenital
sphincter**

Sphincter
urethrae

Compressor
urethrae

Urethrovaginal
sphincter

Vaginal
musculofascial
attachment

Figure 3-2 Components of the urethral supports and sphincteric mechanisms. The proximal urethra and bladder neck are supported by the anterior vaginal wall and its musculofascial attachments to the pelvic diaphragm. The *inset* shows how contraction of the levator ani muscles elevates the anterior vagina, bladder neck, and proximal urethra, contributing to bladder neck closure. The sphincter urethrae, urethrovaginal sphincter, and compressor urethrae all are points of the striated urogenital sphincter.

The bladder is a hollow, muscular organ that is a low-pressure reservoir for the urinary system. The bladder wall musculature is often described as having inner longitudinal, middle circular, and outer longitudinal smooth muscle bundles. However, this layering occurs only at the bladder neck, with the remainder of the bladder musculature composed of fibers that run in many directions. This plexiform arrangement of smooth muscle bundles is ideally suited to allowing the bladder to hold large volumes of urine while maintaining very low pressures and voluntarily contracting when micturition is desired. In a neurologically intact woman, these muscle bundles should work synergistically with the large pelvic floor muscles and the skeletal sphincter mechanisms of the urethra.

The trigone of the bladder is a triangular area in the base of the bladder that is lined with a smooth epithelial covering. The corners of the trigone are formed by the paired ureteral orifices and the internal urethral meatus. The superior boundary of the trigone is a slightly raised area between the two ureteric orifices, called the interureteric ridge. The two ureteral openings are slitlike and lie about 3 cm apart when the bladder is empty.

The pelvic ureter is the portion of the ureter below the level of the ilial vessels. In its lowest portion, it courses along the lateral side of the uterosacral ligament and enters the endopelvic fascia of the parametrium (cardinal ligament). The distal ureter then moves medially over the lateral vaginal fornix and travels through the wall of the bladder until reaching the trigone (**Video 3-2** ; see Figure 3-1).

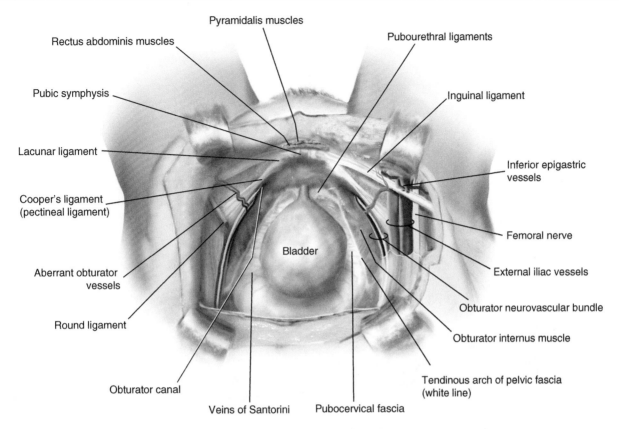

Figure 3-3 Normal anatomy of the pelvis viewed from above. The proximal urethra and extraperitoneal portions of the bladder are exposed through the retropubic space. Note the trapezoid-shaped endopelvic fascia or inside lining of the muscular portion of the vaginal wall. The fascia provides the support for the anterior wall.

(From Baggish MS, Karram MM, eds. Atlas of Pelvic Anatomy and Gynecologic Surgery, *ed 3. St. Louis: Saunders; 2011.)*

Anatomy of the Retropubic Space

The boundaries of the retropubic space (space of Retzius) are the symphysis pubis anteriorly, the pubic rami laterally, and the sidewalls composed of pubic bone and obturator internist muscle. The anterior aspects of the proximal urethra and extraperitoneal portions of the bladder are seen on exposure of the retropubic space. Figure 3-3 illustrates the view from above the retropubic space. The floor of the retropubic space is formed by the fibrofatty outer lining of the vaginal wall termed the endopelvic fascia, the paravesical fascia, and the fibers from the levator ani muscle. This trapezoid-shaped structure provides support for the proximal urethra and bladder. Figure 3-4 shows a sagittal section of the normal anatomy of the pelvis and demonstrates the relationship of the retropubic space to the urinary bladder and pelvic sidewall. There is adipose tissue behind the symphysis pubis, between the bladder and the pubic bone, that can be gently separated by blunt finger dissection. The space progressively develops from the superior to the inferior margin of the pubic symphysis. The lateral development of the retropubic space extends to the paravesical space and terminates at the pelvic sidewall or more precisely at the obturator internus muscle. The arcus tendineus fasciae pelvis originates from the obturator internus fascia. This whitish thickening of the obturator fascia can vary in its configuration from a single line to a wishbone or double-blind structure. The pubococcygeus portion of the levator ani takes its origin from the arcus tendineus. The broad levator ani

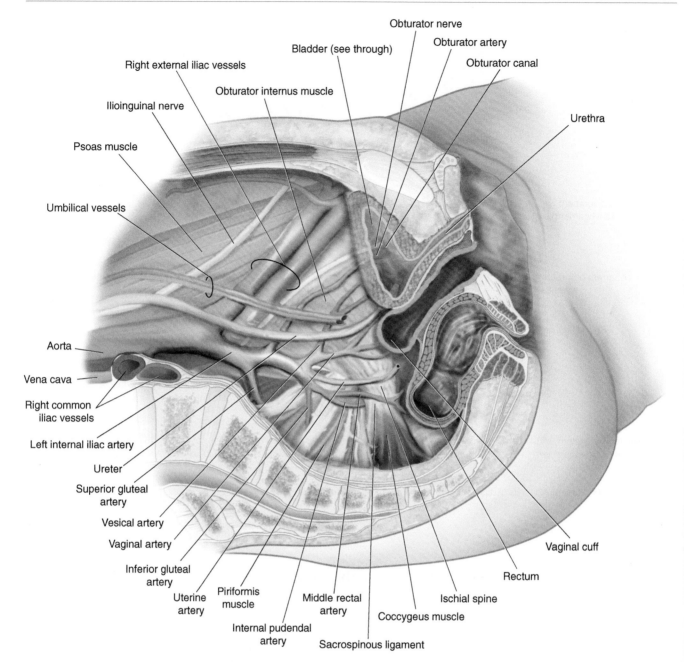

Figure 3-4 Sagittal section of normal anatomy of the pelvis. Note how the various vessels, nerves, and muscles relate to the bladder and retropubic space. The external iliac vessels exit the pelvis underneath the inguinal ligament just lateral to the uppermost portion of the retropubic space, whereas the obturator neurovascular bundle passes through the retropubic space to exit the pelvis through the obturator canal.

(From Baggish MS, Karram MM, eds. Atlas of Pelvic Anatomy and Gynecologic Surgery, *ed 3. St. Louis: Saunders; 2011.)*

funnels downward into the depths of the pelvis. A portion of the levator ani arises from the inferior margin of the pubic ramus on either side in close proximity to the urethra where it plays a key role in the sphincter mechanism required to maintain bladder control and allow normal voiding. At the inferior extent of the space, the urethrovesical junction, the anterior lateral vaginal fornices, and the levator ani muscles are identified (**Videos 3-3** and **3-4**). **Video 3-5** demonstrates important anatomic landmarks in and around the retropubic space related to passage of tension-free vaginal tape trocars.

The urethrovesical junction and the greater mass of the urinary bladder are exposed within the space of Retzius. Specifically, these structures lie on the

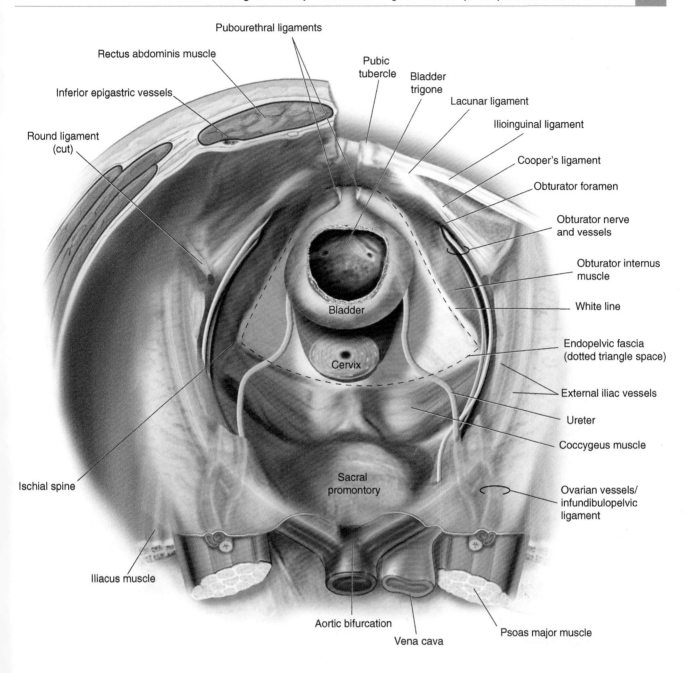

Pubourethral ligaments

Rectus abdominis muscle

Inferior epigastric vessels

Round ligament (cut)

Pubic tubercle

Bladder trigone

Lacunar ligament

Ilioinguinal ligament

Cooper's ligament

Obturator foramen

Obturator nerve and vessels

Obturator internus muscle

White line

Endopelvic fascia (dotted triangle space)

External iliac vessels

Ureter

Coccygeus muscle

Ovarian vessels/ infundibulopelvic ligament

Bladder

Cervix

Sacral promontory

Ischial spine

Iliacus muscle

Aortic bifurcation

Vena cava

Psoas major muscle

Normal Anatomy

Figure 3-5 Surgical anatomy of the retropubic space. The proximal urethra and bladder rest on the anterior vaginal wall with its underlying muscular component, or pubocervical fascia. The vagina attaches laterally to the white line, or arcus tendineus fasciae pelvis. The veins of Santorini run within the vaginal wall and are commonly encountered during colposuspension procedures. Other important vascular structures that may be encountered in this space include the obturator neurovascular bundle, the aberrant obturator artery and vein, and the external iliac artery and vein.

(From Baggish MS, Karram MM, eds. Atlas of Pelvic Anatomy and Gynecologic Surgery, *ed 3. St. Louis: Saunders; 2011.)*

floor of the retropubic space. The pubourethral ligaments are noted at the level of the proximal urethra. These are shown in Figures 3-5 and 3-6. Figure 3-6 also shows the anatomy of the retropubic space as it relates to the thigh. The arcus tendineus fasciae pelvis or white line stretches from the posterior aspect of the symphysis pubis and continues in a downward sloping direction along the fascia margin of the obturator internus muscles to terminate in the ischial

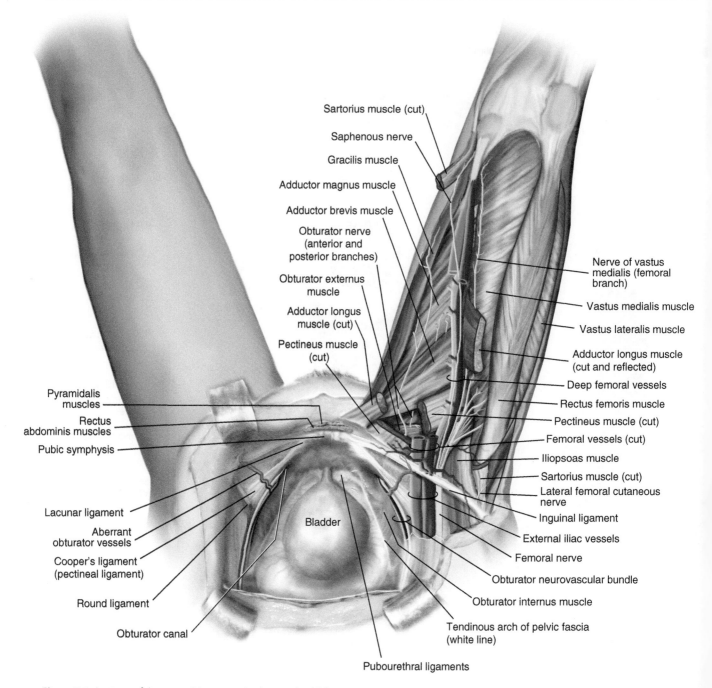

Sartorius muscle (cut)

Saphenous nerve

Gracilis muscle

Adductor magnus muscle

Adductor brevis muscle

Obturator nerve
(anterior and
posterior branches)

Obturator externus
muscle

Adductor longus
muscle (cut)

Pectineus muscle
(cut)

Nerve of vastus
medialis (femoral
branch)

Vastus medialis muscle

Vastus lateralis muscle

Adductor longus muscle
(cut and reflected)

Deep femoral vessels

Rectus femoris muscle

Pectineus muscle (cut)

Femoral vessels (cut)

Iliopsoas muscle

Sartorius muscle (cut)

Lateral femoral cutaneous
nerve

Inguinal ligament

External iliac vessels

Femoral nerve

Obturator neurovascular bundle

Obturator internus muscle

Tendinous arch of pelvic fascia
(white line)

Pyramidalis
muscles

Rectus
abdominis muscles

Pubic symphysis

Lacunar ligament

Aberrant
obturator vessels

Cooper's ligament
(pectineal ligament)

Round ligament

Obturator canal

Bladder

Pubourethral ligaments

Figure 3-6 Anatomy of the retropubic space as it relates to the thigh.

(From Baggish MS, Karram MM, eds. Atlas of Pelvic Anatomy and Gynecologic Surgery, *ed 3. St. Louis: Saunders; 2011.)*

spine. The attachment of the muscular portion of the vaginal wall to the white line maintains the support of the lateral vaginal wall. Detachment of this tissue from the white line leads to a paravaginal defect. The iliococcygeus portion of the levator ani takes its origin from the arcus and swings downward toward the midline composing a portion of pelvic floor. The levator ani muscle envelopes the urethra, vagina, and rectum. If the symphysis pubis is cut in the midline with a saw, the levator ani muscle can be followed inferiorly as it inserts into the lateral walls of the vagina and urethra deep to the vestibular bulb and clitoral crura.

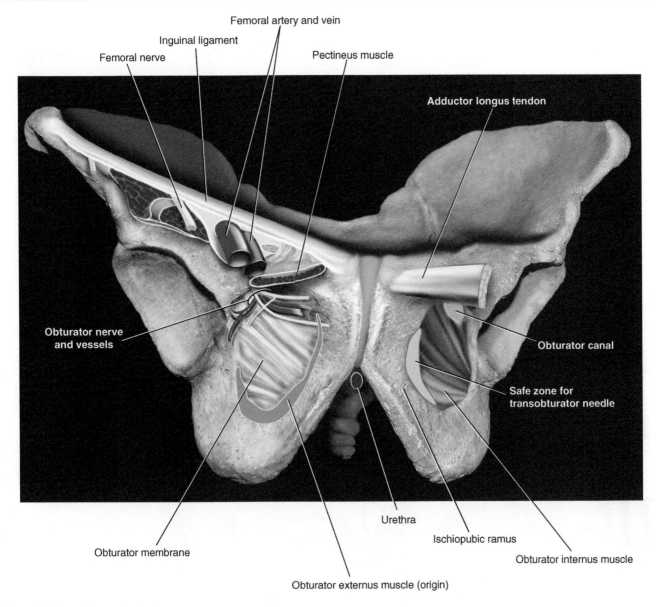

Femoral artery and vein

Inguinal ligament

Femoral nerve

Pectineus muscle

Adductor longus tendon

Obturator nerve
and vessels

Obturator canal

Safe zone for
transobturator needle

Obturator membrane

Urethra

Ischiopubic ramus

Obturator internus muscle

Obturator externus muscle (origin)

Figure 3-7 Transobturator landmarks.

Transobturator Anatomy and Anatomy of the Inner Groin

The obturator membrane is a fibrous sheath that spans the obturator foramen, through which the obturator neurovascular bundle penetrates via the obturator canal. Figure 3-7 shows transobturator landmarks of importance when performing transobturator slings, and **Video 3-6** demonstrates the anatomy of the inner groin as it relates to transobturator sling placement. The obturator artery and vein originate as branches of the internal iliac vessels. As they emerge from the inferior side of the obturator membrane and enter the obturator space, they divide into many small branches supplying the muscles of the adductor compartment of the thigh. Work on cadavers by Whiteside and Walters (2004) has contradicted previous reports of the obturator vessels bifurcating into medial and lateral branches; rather, the vessels are predominantly small (<5 mm in diameter) and splinter into variable courses. The muscles of the medial thigh adductor compartment are, from superficial to deep, the gracilis, adductor longus, adductor brevis, adductor magnus, and obturator externus muscles (Figure 3-8). In contrast to the

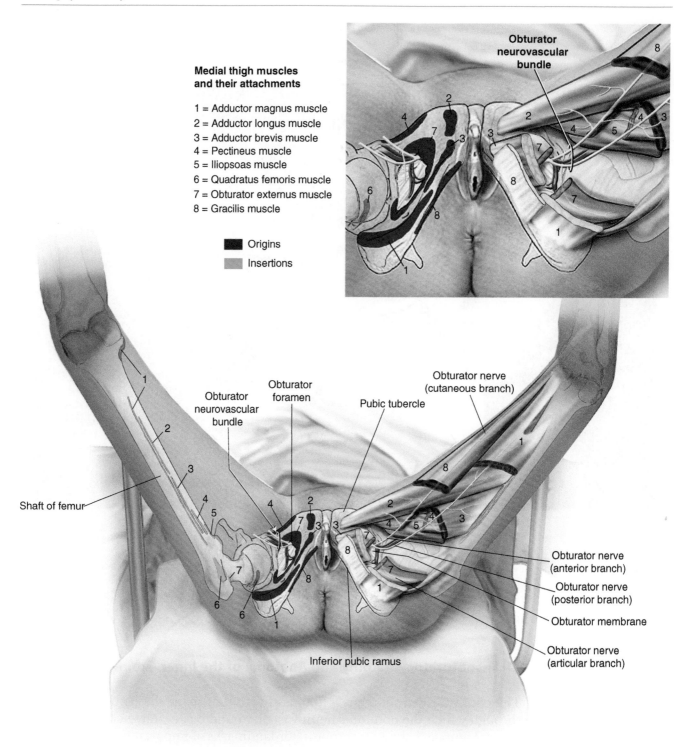

**Medial thigh muscles
and their attachments**

1 = Adductor magnus muscle
2 = Adductor longus muscle
3 = Adductor brevis muscle
4 = Pectineus muscle
5 = Iliopsoas muscle
6 = Quadratus femoris muscle
7 = Obturator externus muscle
8 = Gracilis muscle

■ Origins
■ Insertions

Figure 3-8 Anatomy of the inner thigh. Note the origins and insertions of medial thigh muscles.

(From Baggish MS, Karram MM, eds. Atlas of Pelvic Anatomy and Gynecologic Surgery, *ed 3. St. Louis: Saunders; 2011.)*

vessels, the obturator nerve emerges from the obturator membrane and bifurcates into anterior and posterior divisions traveling distally down the thigh to supply the muscles of the adductor compartment. With the patient in the dorsal lithotomy position, the nerves and vessels of the thigh course laterally away from the tissue of pubis ramus. Figure 3-9 demonstrates the anatomic location of the ischiopubic ramus as it relates to the inner thigh, and Figure 3-10

Figure 3-9 The bony pelvis held in front of a cadaver to demonstrate the anatomic location of the ischiopubic ramus and the obturator foramen.

(From Baggish MS, Karram MM, eds. Atlas of Pelvic Anatomy and Gynecologic Surgery, *ed 3. St. Louis: Saunders; 2011.)*

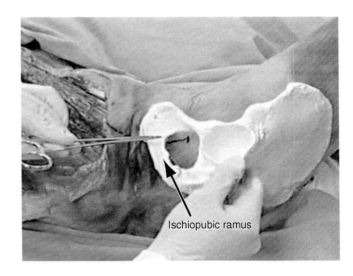

Ischiopubic ramus

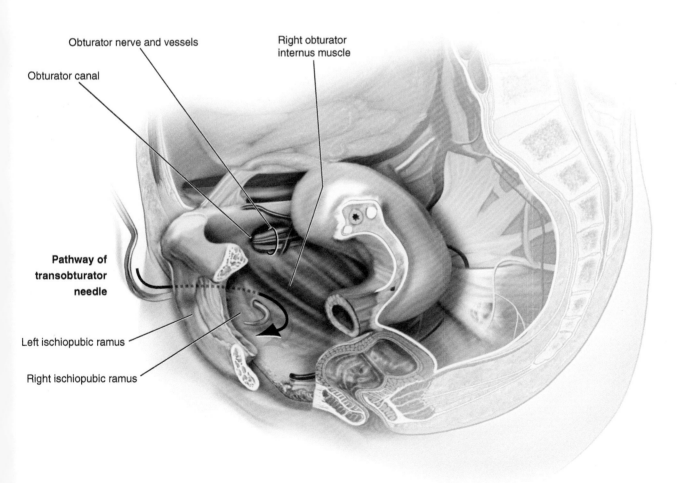

Obturator nerve and vessels

Obturator canal

Right obturator internus muscle

Pathway of transobturator needle

Left ischiopubic ramus

Right ischiopubic ramus

Figure 3-10 Cross section of pelvis demonstrating appropriate path for transobturator needle passage around ischiopubic ramus.

illustrates the appropriate needle entry and path of transobturator needle passage.

Suggested Readings

DeLancey JO. Correlative study of paraurethral anatomy. *Obstet Gynecol.* 1986;68:91.

DeLancey JO. Structural aspects of the extrinsic continence mechanism. *Obstet Gynecol.* 1988;72:296.

DeLancey JO. Pubovesical ligament: a separate structure from the urethral supports ("pubo-urethral ligaments"). *Neurourol Urodyn.* 1989;8:53.

Gosling JA. The structure of the female lower urinary tract and pelvic floor. *Urol Clin North Am.* 1985;12:207.

Gosling JA, Dixon JS, Critchley HO, et al. A comparative study of the human external sphincter and periurethral levator ani muscles. *Br J Urol.* 1981;53:35.

Milley PS, Nichols DH. The relationship between the pubo-urethral ligaments and the urogenital diaphragm in the human female. *Anat Rec.* 1971;170:281.

Nichols DH, Randall CL. *Vaginal Surgery,* ed 3. Baltimore: Williams & Wilkins; 1989.

Oelrich TM. The striated urogenital sphincter muscle in the female. *Anat Rec.* 1983;250:223.

Olesen KP, Grau V. The suspensory apparatus of the female bladder neck. *Urol Int.* 1976;31:33.

Ulmsten U, Petros P. Intravaginal slingplasty (IVS): an ambulatory surgical procedure for treatment of female urinary incontinence. *Scand J Urol Nephrol.* 1995;29(1):75.

Whiteside JL, Walters MD. Anatomy of the obturator region: relations to a transobturator sling. *Int Urogynecol J.* 2004;15:223.

Retropubic Operations for Stress Urinary Incontinence

4

Mark D. Walters, M.D.

 Videos

4-1 Modified Burch Colposuspension   **4-2** Laparoscopic Paravaginal Repair

Introduction

Since 1949, when Marshall et al. first described retropubic urethrovesical suspension for the treatment of stress urinary incontinence (SUI), retropubic procedures have proved to be consistently curative. Although numerous terminologies and variations of retropubic repairs have been described, the basic goal remains the same: to suspend and to stabilize the anterior vaginal wall, and with it the bladder neck and proximal urethra, in a retropubic position. This suspension prevents the descent of these structures and allows urethral compression against a stable suburethral layer. Selection of a retropubic approach (vs. a vaginal approach) depends on many factors, such as the need for laparotomy or laparoscopy for other pelvic prolapse or disease, amount of pelvic organ prolapse, status of the intrinsic urethral sphincter mechanism, age and health status of the patient, history of previous sling or mesh complications, desires of future fertility, preference and expertise of the surgeon, and preferences of an informed patient.

Historically, there were few data to differentiate one retropubic procedure from another. The three most studied and popular retropubic procedures were the Burch colposuspension, the Marshall-Marchetti-Krantz (MMK) procedure, and the paravaginal defect repair. I prefer the Burch colposuspension for urodynamic SUI with bladder neck hypermobility and adequate resting urethral sphincter function, and sometimes combine it with a paravaginal defect repair when the patient has stage 2 or 3 anterior vaginal prolapse or when a concurrent sacrocolpopexy is to be done. The surgical techniques described in this chapter are contemporary modifications of the original operations. Tanagho (1976) described the modified Burch colposuspension. The paravaginal defect repair was described by Richardson et al. (1981) and Shull and Baden (1989) (paravaginal repair) and by Turner-Warwick (1986) and Webster and Kreder (1990) (vaginal obturator shelf repair). Although less critically studied, the paravaginal defect repair, until more recently, was regionally popular and widely performed in the United States. The operations described do not represent one correct technique but a commonly used and proven method.

This chapter describes only retropubic suspension procedures that use an abdominal wall incision for direct access into the space of Retzius. The use of laparoscopy and mini-incision laparotomy to enter the retropubic space and perform these and similar procedures is possible and occasionally preferred. The decision to use laparoscopy and mini-incision laparotomy usually is based on whether other concurrent surgeries need to be done and on what is most desired by the surgeon and the informed patient. The reader is referred to *Surgical Management of Pelvic Organ Prolapse* (Karram and Maher, 2012) in the Female Pelvic Surgery Video Atlas series for a thorough critique of the use of operative laparoscopy for urinary incontinence and prolapse.

Case 1: Stress Urinary Incontinence and Large Uterine Fibroids

A 46-year-old, para 3 woman complains of heavy painful menstrual periods, pelvic pressure, and bothersome urine loss with coughing and exercise. She states that she has been diagnosed with uterine fibroids in the past, but her symptoms are worse this year. Pelvic examination reveals a 16-week-size globular mobile uterus and no other pelvic masses. On vaginal examination, she has stage 1 anterior vaginal wall prolapse with urethral hypermobility. She has no uterine or posterior vaginal wall prolapse and good levator muscle function during voluntary pelvic muscle squeeze. She has no history of abnormal Papanicolaou (Pap) smears and had a normal Pap test and human papillomavirus screen 1 year earlier. On office urodynamics evaluation, she is examined with a full bladder in the supine position and noted to leak urine with coughing from the urethra. She voided 360 mL and had a catheterized post-void residual urine volume of 20 mL. Her urinalysis is negative.

Discussion of treatment options includes conservative and medical management of uterine fibroids and menorrhagia and conservative management with physical therapy for SUI. She states that she has been bothered by both problems for many years, has previously not improved with hormone therapy and Kegel exercises, and is now interested in definitive therapy including a hysterectomy. She also notes that she would prefer not to have mesh placed during the reconstructive surgery unless absolutely necessary.

After discussing all of the options for routes of hysterectomy and for treatment of SUI, it was decided that the patient would undergo an open total abdominal hysterectomy, Burch colposuspension, and cystoscopy using a Pfannenstiel incision. After the hysterectomy was completed, she would have reattachment of her uterosacral ligaments to the vaginal cuff. This treatment was accomplished without complication.

Indications for Retropubic Procedures

Retropubic urethrovesical suspension procedures are indicated for women with a diagnosis of urodynamic SUI and a hypermobile proximal urethra and bladder neck. Although midurethral slings are usually performed as first-line surgical treatment for these patients, Burch colposuspension remains an option because studies have shown similar efficacy to slings. In patients who do not wish to have surgery that uses synthetic mesh, Burch colposuspension and fascial slings are the best options. Retropubic procedures usually are not used for intrinsic sphincter deficiency with urethral hypermobility because other, more obstructive operations such as a retropubic bladder neck or midurethral sling are likely to yield better long-term results.

To diagnose urodynamic SUI, clinical and urodynamics (simple or complex) testing must be performed to evaluate bladder filling, storage, and emptying (see Chapter 2). Abnormalities of bladder-filling function, such as detrusor overactivity, can coexist with urethral sphincter incompetence in 30% of patients and may be associated with a lower cure rate after retropubic surgery.

Women with SUI generally should have a trial of conservative therapy before corrective surgery is offered. Conservative treatments include pelvic muscle exercises, bladder retraining, pharmacologic therapy, and mechanical devices such as pessaries. Eligible and willing postmenopausal patients with atrophic urogenital changes should be prescribed vaginal estrogen before surgery is considered.

Surgical Techniques

Operative Setup and General Entry into the Retropubic Space

1. The patient is supine, with the legs supported in a slightly abducted position, allowing the surgeon to operate with one hand in the vagina and the other in the retropubic space. The vagina, perineum, and abdomen are sterilely prepared and draped in a fashion that permits easy access to the lower abdomen and vagina.

2. A three-way 16F or 20F Foley catheter with a 20- to 30-mL balloon is inserted in a sterile fashion into the bladder and kept in the sterile field. The drainage port of the catheter is left to gravity drainage, and the irrigation port is connected to sterile water with or without blue dye.

3. One perioperative intravenous dose of an appropriate antibiotic should be given as prophylaxis against infection within 1 hour before the incision is made.

4. A Pfannenstiel incision is usually the preferred type of skin incision. Entrance into the retropubic space sometimes may be facilitated by using a Cherney incision (Figure 4-1). During intraperitoneal surgery, the peritoneum is opened, the surgery is completed, and the cul-de-sac is plicated, if necessary.

5. The retropubic space is exposed. Staying close to the back of the pubic bone, the surgeon's hand is introduced into the retropubic space and the bladder and urethra are gently moved downward (Figure 4-2). Sharp dissection usually is not necessary in primary cases. To aid visualization of the bladder, 100 mL of sterile water with methylene blue or indigo carmine dye may be instilled into the bladder after the catheter drainage port is clamped.

6. If previous retropubic or other bladder neck suspension procedures have been performed, dense adhesions from the anterior vaginal and bladder wall and urethra to the symphysis pubis are often present. These adhesions should be dissected sharply from the pubic bone until the anterior bladder wall, urethra, and vagina are free of adhesions and are mobile. If identification of the urethra or lower border of the bladder is difficult, one may perform a cystotomy, which, with a finger inside the bladder, helps to define the lower limits of the bladder for easier dissection, mobilization, and elevation (Figure 4-3).

Technique for Burch Colposuspension (Video 4-1 📹)

1. After the retropubic space is entered, the urethra and anterior vaginal wall are depressed. No dissection should be performed in the midline over the urethra or at the urethrovesical junction, protecting the delicate musculature of the urethra from surgical trauma. Attention is directed to the tissue on either side of the urethra. The surgeon's nondominant hand is placed in the vagina, palm facing upward, with the index and middle fingers on each side of the proximal urethra. Most of the overlying fat should be cleared away, using a swab mounted on a curved forceps sponge stick. This dissection is accomplished with forceful elevation of the surgeon's vaginal finger until

Figure 4-1 Technique of performing a Cherney incision to facilitate entrance into the retropubic space. **A,** The rectus muscle is isolated and exposed very low near its insertion into the pubic bone. **B,** Monopolar cautery is used to cut through the lowest portion of the rectus muscle. **C,** The rectus muscle is reflected back, allowing easy access to the retropubic space. If the peritoneum is going to be entered, it should be opened with a transverse incision.

(From Baggish MS, Karram MM, eds. Atlas of Pelvic Anatomy and Gynecology Surgery, *ed 3. St. Louis: Saunders; 2011.)*

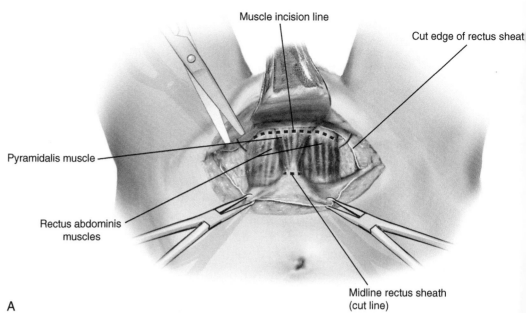

Muscle incision line

Cut edge of rectus sheath

Pyramidalis muscle

Rectus abdominis muscles

Midline rectus sheath (cut line)

A

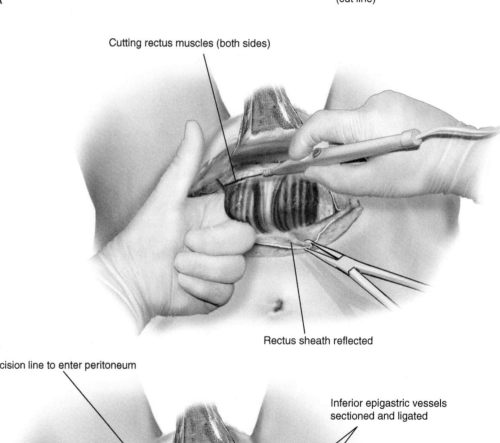

Cutting rectus muscles (both sides)

Rectus sheath reflected

B

Incision line to enter peritoneum

Inferior epigastric vessels sectioned and ligated

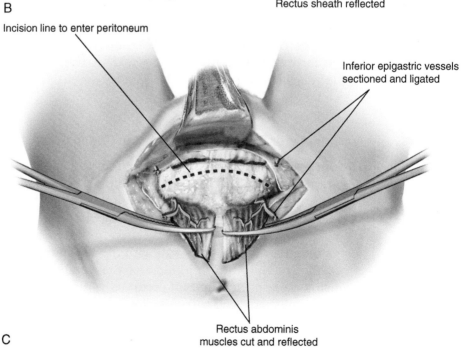

Rectus abdominis muscles cut and reflected

C

Figure 4-2 Technique used to expose the retropubic space. The surgeon's hand is used to gently displace the bladder and urethra downward.

(From Baggish MS, Karram MM, eds. Atlas of Pelvic Anatomy and Gynecology Surgery, *ed 3. St. Louis: Saunders; 2011.)*

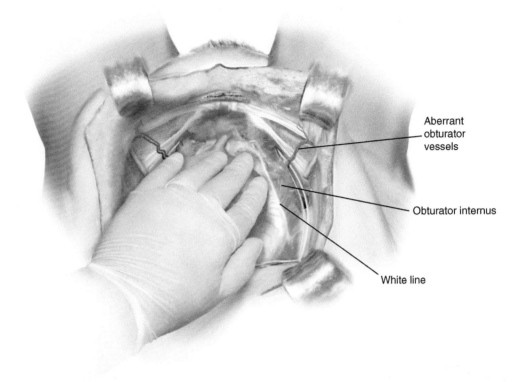

Aberrant obturator vessels

Obturator internus

White line

Figure 4-3 Retropubic vesicourethrolysis. A high extraperitoneal cystotomy has been made to facilitate sharp dissection of the bladder from the back of the symphysis pubis.

(From Baggish MS, Karram MM, eds. Atlas of Pelvic Anatomy and Gynecology Surgery, *ed 3. St. Louis: Saunders; 2011.)*

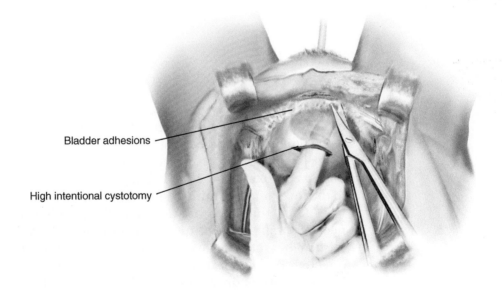

Bladder adhesions

High intentional cystotomy

glistening white periurethral fascia and vaginal wall are seen (Figure 4-4). This area is extremely vascular, with a rich, thin-walled venous plexus that should be avoided, if possible. The position of the urethra and the lower edge of the bladder is determined by palpating the Foley balloon and by partially distending the bladder to define the rounded lower margin of the bladder as it meets the anterior vaginal wall.

2. When dissection lateral to the urethra is completed and vaginal mobility is judged to be adequate by using the vaginal fingers to lift the anterior vaginal wall upward and forward, sutures are placed. No. 0 or 1 delayed absorbable or nonabsorbable sutures are placed as far laterally in the anterior vaginal

Figure 4-4 Burch colposuspension. The bladder is gently mobilized to the opposite side with sponge sticks. The anterior vaginal wall is elevated by the middle finger of the surgeon's nondominant hand, and fat is mobilized medially (see *inset*) with a swab mounted on a curved forceps or suction tip. The position of the sutures (indicated with *X*) ideally should be at least 2 cm lateral to the proximal urethra and bladder neck, usually on the lateral downslope of the tissue elevated by the vaginal finger.

(From Baggish MS, Karram MM, eds. Atlas of Pelvic Anatomy and Gynecology Surgery, *ed 3. St. Louis: Saunders; 2011.)*

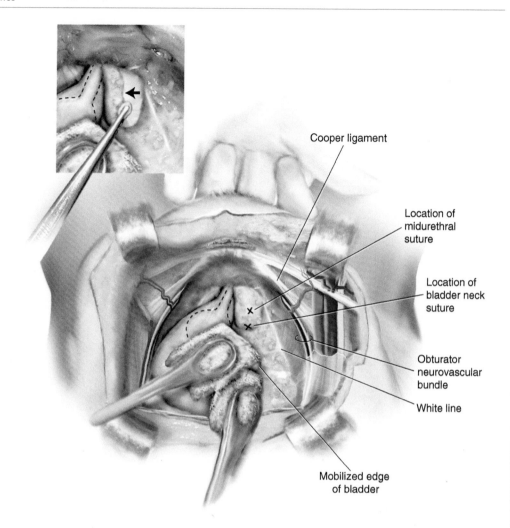

wall as is technically possible. We apply two sutures of No. 0 braided polyester on an SH needle (Ethibond; Ethicon, Inc, Somerville, NJ) bilaterally, using double bites for each suture. The distal suture is placed approximately 2 cm lateral to the proximal third of the urethra. The proximal suture is placed approximately 2 cm lateral to the bladder wall at or slightly proximal to the level of the urethrovesical junction. In placing the sutures, one should take a full thickness of vaginal wall, excluding the epithelium, with the needle parallel to the urethra (Figure 4-5). This maneuver is best accomplished by suturing over the surgeon's vaginal finger at the appropriate selected sites. On each side, after the two sutures are placed, they are passed through the pectineal (Cooper) ligament so that all four suture ends exit above the ligament. Before the sutures are tied, a 1 × 4 cm strip of absorbable gelatin sponge (Gelfoam) may be placed between the vagina and obturator fascia below the Cooper ligament to aid adherence and hemostasis.

3. As noted previously, this area is extremely vascular, and visible vessels should be avoided if possible. When excessive bleeding occurs, it can be controlled by direct pressure, sutures, or vascular clips. Less severe bleeding usually stops with direct pressure and after tying the suspension sutures.

4. After all four sutures are placed in the vagina and through the Cooper ligaments, the assistant ties first the distal sutures and then the proximal ones, while the surgeon elevates the vagina with the vaginal hand. In tying the sutures, one does not have to be concerned about whether the vaginal wall

Figure 4-5 Sutures have been appropriately placed on each side of the proximal urethral and bladder neck. Figure-of-eight bites are taken through the vagina. Double-armed sutures are used so that the end of each suture can be brought up through the ipsilateral Cooper ligament, allowing the sutures to be tied above the ligament.

(From Baggish MS, Karram MM, eds. Atlas of Pelvic Anatomy and Gynecology Surgery, *ed 3. St. Louis: Saunders; 2011.)*

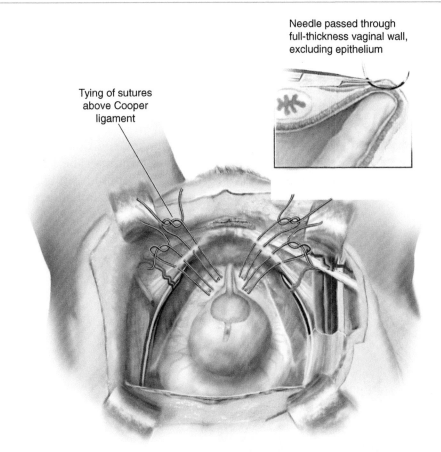

Tying of sutures above Cooper ligament

Needle passed through full-thickness vaginal wall, excluding epithelium

meets the Cooper ligament, so one should not place too much tension on the vaginal wall. A suture bridge is usually found between the two points. After the sutures are tied, one can easily insert two fingers between the pubic bone and the urethra, preventing compression of the urethra against the pubic bone. Vaginal fixation and urethral support depend more on fibrosis and scarring of periurethral and vaginal tissues over the obturator internus and levator fascia than on the suture material itself (see **Video 6-1**).

Paravaginal Defect Repair (Video 4-2)

The object of the paravaginal defect repair is to reattach, bilaterally, the anterolateral vaginal sulcus with its overlying endopelvic fascia to the pubococcygeus and obturator internus muscles and fascia at the level of the arcus tendineus fasciae pelvis.

1. The retropubic space is entered, and the bladder and vagina are depressed and pulled medially to allow visualization of the lateral retropubic space, including the obturator internus and levator muscles, and the fossa containing the obturator neurovascular bundle.

2. Blunt dissection can be carried dorsally from this point until the ischial spine is palpated. The arcus tendineus fasciae pelvis is often visualized as a white band of tissue running over the pubococcygeus and obturator internus muscles from the back of the lower edge of the symphysis pubis toward the ischial spine. A lateral paravaginal defect representing avulsion of the vagina off the arcus tendineus fasciae pelvis or of the arcus tendineus fasciae pelvis off the obturator internus muscle may be visualized.

3. The surgeon's nondominant hand is inserted into the vagina. While gently retracting the vagina and bladder medially, the surgeon elevates the antero-lateral vaginal sulcus. Starting near the vaginal apex, a suture is placed, first through the full thickness of the vagina (excluding the vaginal epithelium) and then deep into the obturator internus fascia or arcus tendineus fasciae pelvis, 1 to 2 cm anterior to its origin at the ischial spine. After this first stitch is tied, additional (three to five) sutures are placed through the vaginal wall and overlying fascia and then into the obturator internus at about 1-cm intervals toward the pubic ramus. The most distal sutures should be placed as close as possible to the pubic ramus, into the pubourethral ligament (Figure 4-6). Burch colposuspension sutures can be placed bilaterally at the

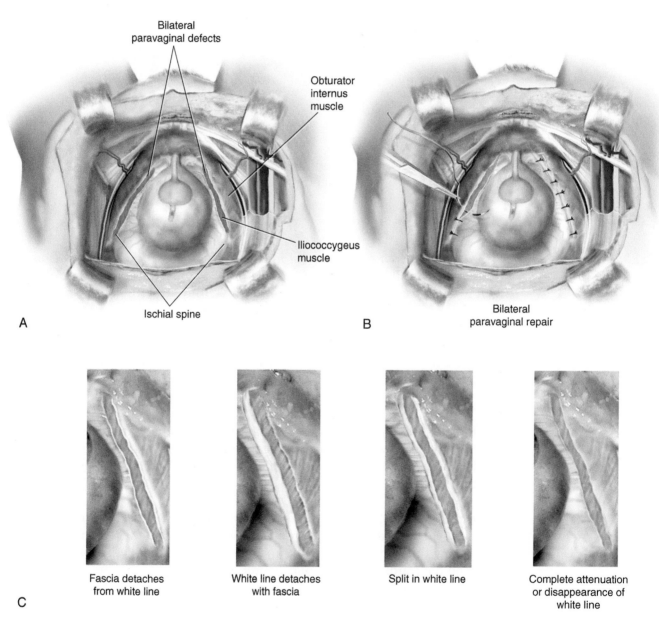

Figure 4-6 Retropubic paravaginal defect repair. **A,** Bilateral paravaginal defects are illustrated. **B,** The defect on the right has been completely repaired, and the defect on the left is being repaired from just distal to the ischial spine and working toward the pubic symphysis. **C,** Four potential anatomic findings in patients with paravaginal defects are illustrated. All anatomic findings result in falling away of the vagina with its underlying fasciae from the lateral pelvic sidewall.

(From Baggish MS, Karram MM, eds. Atlas of Pelvic Anatomy and Gynecology Surgery, *ed 3. St. Louis: Saunders; 2011.)*

level of the bladder neck and urethra if the patient has SUI. No. 2-0 or 0 nonabsorbable suture on a medium-sized, tapered needle usually is used for the paravaginal repair (Figure 4-7).

This procedure leaves free space between the symphysis pubis and the proximal urethra but secure support so that rotational descent of the proximal urethra and bladder base is prevented with sudden increases in intraabdominal pressure. According to Turner-Warwick (1986), it avoids overcorrection and fixation of the periurethral fascia, which might compromise the functional movements of the urethra and bladder base and lead to obstruction and voiding difficulty. This principle may explain why the paravaginal defect repair usually results in spontaneous voiding on the first or second postoperative day. The vaginal obturator shelf repair was used to correct patients with dysfunctional voiding symptoms after previous retropubic surgery.

General Intraoperative and Postoperative Procedures

If the surgeon is concerned that intravesical suture placement or ureteral obstruction may have occurred, cystoscopy—either transurethrally or through the dome of the bladder—or a small cystotomy may be performed to document ureteral patency and absence of intravesical sutures after retropubic procedures. Intravenous injection of indigo carmine before cystoscopy aids visualization of urine from the ureters.

Closed suction drains in the retropubic space are used only as necessary when hemostasis is incomplete and there is concern about postoperative hematoma. The bladder is routinely drained with a suprapubic or transurethral catheter for 1 to 2 days. After that time, the patient is allowed to begin voiding trials, and post-void residual urine volumes are checked, either with the suprapubic catheter or by intermittent self-catheterization.

Figure 4-7 Paravaginal defect plus repair. Combined Burch colposuspension and retropubic paravaginal defect repair.

(From Baggish MS, Karram MM, eds. Atlas of Pelvic Anatomy and Gynecology Surgery, *ed 3. St. Louis: Saunders; 2011.)*

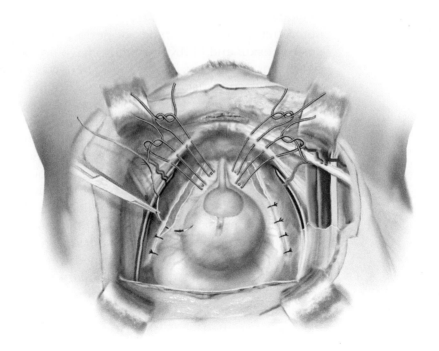

Outcomes

Many studies have reported clinical experiences with retropubic urethral suspension procedures for SUI. Quality studies, including prospective randomized trials, have been conducted comparing Burch colposuspension with synthetic midurethral and pubovaginal fascial slings. Only a few studies have assessed the paravaginal defect repair for SUI. Early studies using subjective outcome measures reported that greater than 90% of women were continent after this procedure. However, in a prospective randomized trial, Columbo et al. (1996) found that only 61% of women were continent 3 years after a paravaginal defect repair compared with 100% of women continent after a Burch colposuspension. We currently believe that the paravaginal defect repair should be used only selectively for anatomic correction of anterior vaginal wall prolapse and not as primary treatment of SUI.

Multiple studies with objective measures of cure reported that the Burch colposuspension is effective for women with urodynamically proved SUI. At 3 to 24 months after surgery, 59% to 100% of patients become continent, for an overall average cure rate of about 85%. At 3 to 7 years, continence rates range from 63% to 89%, for an average rate of 77%. Although objectively incontinent, a small percentage of additional patients are improved and satisfied with their surgical results. The overall reported absolute failure rate is about 14% at 5 to 7 years.

Eriksen et al. (1990) reported 91 women with urodynamically proved SUI, with or without overactive bladder, who had undergone a Burch colposuspension. After 5 years, 76 patients underwent urodynamics evaluation. Stress incontinence was cured in 71% of the patients with stable bladders preoperatively and in 57% of patients with mixed stress incontinence and detrusor overactivity, a nonsignificant difference. After 5 years, only 52% of the study group was completely dry and free of complications; about 30% needed further incontinence therapy.

Black and Downs published a systematic review in 1996 describing the effectiveness of surgery for SUI in women. The methodologic quality of studies was assessed, including all of the randomized controlled trials to that time. Only two randomized controlled trials of colposuspension were available. The study noted that different methods of performing colposuspension (e.g., Burch colposuspension and MMK procedure) have not been shown to be associated with significant differences in outcome. There was preliminary evidence that laparoscopic colposuspension and open paravaginal defect repair may have lower cure rates than open Burch procedures. Colposuspension appeared to be more effective than anterior colporrhaphy and needle urethropexy procedures in curing and improving SUI. About 85% of women can expect to be continent 1 year after colposuspension compared with 50% to 70% after anterior colporrhaphy and needle suspension. Primary procedures are generally more effective than repeat procedures. The benefit of Burch colposuspension is maintained for at least 5 years, whereas the benefits from anterior colporrhaphy and needle suspension diminish quite rapidly. Of the four prospective studies (done before 1996) comparing Burch colposuspension and sling procedures, none reported a difference in cure, however defined, regardless of whether the operations were performed as primary or secondary operations.

Several studies assessed women more than 10 years after undergoing a Burch procedure. Alcalay et al. (1995) followed a cohort of 109 women (of a group of 366 eligible women) who underwent Burch colposuspension between 1974 and

1983. The mean follow-up interval was 13.8 years. Both subjective and objective outcome measures were collected during the follow-up period. The cure of incontinence was found to be time-dependent, with a decline for 10 to 12 years and then a plateau at 69%. Cure rates were significantly lower in women who had had previous bladder neck surgery. Approximately 10% of patients required at least one additional surgery to cure SUI.

In the first prospective multicenter randomized trial of open Burch colposuspension and tension-free vaginal tape (TVT) for urodynamic stress incontinence, Ward and Hilton (2002) found no significant difference between the surgeries in objective cure rates. Bladder injury was more common during the TVT procedure; delayed voiding, operation time, and return to normal activity all were longer after colposuspension. When these authors analyzed their data at 2 years and ignored subject withdrawals, no differences were seen between the procedures, with objective cure rates of 81% for TVT and 80% for colposuspension (Ward and Hilton, 2004). Jelovsek et al. (2008) reported that laparoscopic Burch colposuspension also had long-term efficacy similar to the TVT sling after a follow-up period of 4 to 8 years.

In 2007, Albo et al., representing the Urinary Incontinence Treatment Network, published a definitive multicenter randomized clinical trial comparing Burch colposuspension with autologous rectus fascia pubovaginal sling. There were 655 women randomly assigned and followed for 24 months. Cure rates of SUI were higher for women who underwent Burch colposuspension (66% vs. 49%; $P < .001$). However, more women who underwent the sling procedure had complications, including urinary tract infections, voiding dysfunction, and postoperative urge incontinence.

A Cochrane review concluded that open Burch colposuspension is effective for SUI especially in the long-term (Lapitan et al., 2009). Continence rates at 1 year were approximately 85% to 90% and at 5 years were about 70%. In 2010, Novara et al. published an updated systematic review and meta-analysis of the comparative data on colposuspensions compared with all slings. These authors concluded that patients treated with retropubic midurethral slings experienced slightly higher continence rates than patients treated with Burch colposuspension, but bladder perforations were more common with retropubic slings.

For years, Burch colposuspension was the antiincontinence procedure of choice in women having an open abdominal sacrocolpopexy (ASC); there has been a recent reevaluation of this both for women with clinical or occult SUI and for women who are continent. Brubaker et al. (2008) showed improved continence rates if a Burch colposuspension was done with ASC whether or not the patient had preoperative SUI. This advantage of adding the Burch procedure to ASC has not been universally reported, however, so the use of prophylactic antiincontinence procedures at ASC remains controversial. Midurethral slings are now frequently combined with ASC to treat clinical and occult SUI. A cohort study from Korea (Moon et al., 2011) showed that transobturator sling resulted in higher cure rates and better functional outcomes than Burch colposuspension with ASC.

Clinical conditions that increase the risk of surgical failure for retropubic colposuspension are listed in Table 4-1 and include baseline urge symptoms, obesity, menopause, prior hysterectomy, prior antiincontinence procedures, and more advanced prolapse. Advanced age and concomitant hysterectomy do not appear to be associated with lower rates of cure after colposuspension. Findings on urodynamics that increase the risk of surgical failure include signs of intrinsic urethral sphincter deficiency, abnormal perineal electromyography,

Table 4–1 Conditions that decrease the chance of cure of incontinence after retropubic colposuspension

Clinical	Urodynamic	Surgical
Greater baseline urge incontinent symptoms	Detrusor overactivity (preoperative or postoperative)	Intraoperative blood loss >1000 mL
Hypoestrogenic state—not on hormone replacement therapy	Intrinsic urethral sphincter deficiency	Concurrent abdominal sacrocolpopexy (?)
Obesity	Lower maximal urethral pressure	
Prior hysterectomy	Lower leak point pressure	
Prior procedures to correct SUI	Lower functional urethral length	
More advanced prolapse	Open bladder neck at rest on videourodynamics	
	Nonmobile bladder neck	
	Abnormal perineal electromyography	

SUI, Stress urinary incontinence.

and concurrent overactive bladder. Patients with intrinsic sphincter deficiency probably are better treated with a more obstructive operation, such as a sling procedure if the urethra is hypermobile or with urethral injections of a bulking agent if the urethra is nonmobile.

Detrusor overactivity or urge incontinence may coexist in 30% of patients with urodynamic SUI. The term "mixed urinary incontinence" has been used to describe this condition. In addition, about 15% of patients with urodynamic SUI who preoperatively have a stable cystometrogram develop de novo detrusor overactivity after a colposuspension procedure. The course of the overactive bladder after a retropubic repair in patients with mixed incontinence is unpredictable. Some studies show that 50% to 60% of patients with mixed incontinence are cured of overactive bladder by surgical support of the bladder neck. A much smaller percentage (approximately 5% to 10%) have worsening of urgency, with the remainder (20% to 30%) having persistence. No preoperative urodynamic parameters have been identified that can accurately predict the course of overactive bladder after incontinence surgery. For this reason, we believe that women with mixed incontinence should initially receive nonsurgical therapy. Karram and Bhatia (1989) found that 32% of women with mixed incontinence became continent after nonsurgical therapy. These data suggest that initial nonsurgical therapy would save one third of patients the cost and morbidity of incontinence surgery.

Complications

Short-Term Postoperative Complications

In a thorough review of the literature, Mainprize and Drutz (1988) summarized the postoperative complications (excluding urinary retention) of open MMK procedures (Table 4-2). Wound complications and urinary infections are the most common surgical complications. Direct surgical injury to the urinary tract occurs rarely. Bladder lacerations occurred in 0.7% of patients; sutures through the bladder and urethra and catheters sewn into the urethra occurred in 0.3% of patients. Ureteral obstruction occurred in 0.1% of patients. Accidental placement of sutures into the bladder during Burch colposuspension or paravaginal defect repair, resulting in vesical stone formation, painful voiding, recurrent cystitis, or fistula, can occur but is rare.

Table 4–2 Postoperative complications in 2712 Marshall-Marchetti-Krantz procedures

Type of Complication	%
Wound, total	5.5
Infection or hematoma	3.4
Hernia or dehiscence	1.8
Urinary tract infection	3.9
Osteitis pubis	2.5
Direct surgical injury to urinary tract	1.6
Bladder tears	0.7
Urethral obstruction	0.5
Sutures through bladder or urethra with or without catheter sewn in	0.3
Ureteral obstruction or hydronephrosis	0.1
Fistula	0.3
Death	0.2

Modified from Mainprize TC, Drutz HP. The Marshall-Marchetti-Krantz procedure: a critical review. *Obstet Gynecol Surv.* 1988;43:724.

Ureteral obstruction occurs rarely after Burch colposuspension and results from ureteral stretching or kinking after elevation of the vagina and bladder base. One study reported three unilateral ureteral obstructions and three bilateral ureteral obstructions in 483 Burch colposuspensions (1.2%). All patients were treated successfully with removal of sutures and ureteral stent placement. No cases of transected ureters have been reported. Ericksen et al. (1990) found that 1 of 75 patients (1.3%) followed for 5 years after Burch procedures had absent unilateral renal function caused by presumed complete ureteral obstruction. This patient had developed only transient postoperative fever.

Lower urinary tract fistulas are uncommon after retropubic procedures, with various types occurring after 0.3% of MMK procedures. Fistulas are probably less common after Burch and paravaginal defect repairs because the sutures are placed several centimeters lateral to the urethra.

Postoperative Voiding Difficulties

The incidence of voiding difficulties after colposuspension varies widely, although patients rarely have urinary retention after 30 days. At my institution, the mean number of days to complete voiding after an open Burch procedure is 7 days. Ericksen et al. (1990) found that only 2 of 91 patients had delayed spontaneous micturition after Burch colposuspension when the catheter was removed the third postoperative day. Of these patients, 15% had residual urine volumes of 100 to 300 mL 5 days after surgery.

Colposuspension can change the original micturition pattern and introduce an element of obstruction that can disturb the balance between voiding forces and outflow resistance, resulting in immediate postoperative and late voiding difficulties. Findings on urodynamics that may occur after colposuspension include decreased flow rate, increased detrusor pressure at maximal flow, and increased urethral resistance.

Urodynamics tests may be used to predict early postoperative voiding difficulties, although their predictive value has not been demonstrated consistently. Bhatia and Bergman (1986) found that all patients with adequate detrusor contraction and flow rates preoperatively were able to resume spontaneous voiding by the seventh postoperative day after Burch colposuspension. One third of patients who voided without detrusor contraction required bladder drainage for 7 days or longer. No patients with decreased flow rates and absent detrusor contraction during voiding were able to void in less than 7 days postoperatively. These authors believed that use of a Valsalva maneuver during voiding may further lead to postoperative voiding difficulties, perhaps by intensifying obstruction at the bladder neck. In a study by Kobak et al. (2001), risk factors for prolonged voiding after Burch colposuspension included advanced age, previous incontinence surgery, increased first sensation to void, high post-void residual volume, and postoperative cystitis. Abdominal straining during voiding was not associated with prolonged voiding after surgery.

Overactive Bladder

Overactive bladder is a recognized postoperative complication of retropubic procedures. Detrusor overactivity as demonstrated on cystometrogram has been reported in 7% to 27% of patients with urodynamic SUI and stable bladders preoperatively, with follow-up of up to 5 years after Burch colposuspension. Postoperative overactive bladder is more common in patients with previous bladder neck surgery and in patients with mixed detrusor overactivity and urodynamic SUI preoperatively. In a study of 148 patients with urodynamic SUI and stable bladders preoperatively, Steel et al. (1986) reported that 24 (16.2%) patients had postoperative detrusor overactivity on cystometrogram 6 months after surgery. Of the 24 patients with overactive bladder, 10 were completely asymptomatic. Of the 14 symptomatic patients, 4 were improved with drugs aimed at correcting the urgency. The remaining 10 patients (6.8%) remained symptomatic with overactive bladder 3 to 5 years after surgery.

The mechanism for this phenomenon is unknown. As noted previously, excessive urethral elevation or compression can lead to partial outflow obstruction and resulting urgency. Whatever the mechanism, postoperative overactive bladder predictably occurs in a small but significant number of patients. Patients undergoing retropubic urethropexy should understand that the operation may cause urgency and urge incontinence, even if it cures their stress incontinence.

Osteitis Pubis

Osteitis pubis is a painful inflammation of periosteum, bone, cartilage, and ligaments of structures of the anterior pelvic girdle. It is a recognized postoperative complication of urologic and radical gynecologic procedures involving the prostate gland or urinary bladder. In urogynecology, osteitis pubis occurs after 0.74% to 2.5% of MMK procedures and only rarely after Burch procedures; the incidence is partially related to the diagnostic criteria used. It also can occur rarely after placement of artificial urinary sphincters and after radical pelvic surgery for gynecologic malignancies.

The cause of osteitis pubis is unclear. It may result from infection, trauma to the periosteum, or impaired circulation in the vessels around the symphysis pubis. The disease typically occurs 2 to 12 weeks postoperatively. Osteitis pubis is characterized by suprapubic pain radiating to the thighs and is exacerbated by walking or abduction of the lower extremities, marked tenderness and swelling over the symphysis pubis, and radiographic evidence of bone destruction with separation of the symphysis pubis. The clinical course varies from prolonged, progressive debilitation over several months to spontaneous resolution after several weeks. Suggested conservative treatments include rest, physical therapy, steroids, and nonsteroidal antiinflammatory agents. Whatever the therapy, however, noninfectious osteitis pubis tends to be self-limiting.

Recalcitrant cases of osteitis pubis may be due to pubic osteomyelitis. Diagnosis is made by bone biopsy and bacterial culture. Kammerer-Doak et al. (1998) found positive cultures in 71% of patients with clinical osteitis pubis who failed to respond to conservative therapy. Treatments are antibiotics, incision and drainage if abscess formation occurs, or symphyseal wedge resection or débridement.

Enterocele and Rectocele

Burch (1968) first reported that enteroceles occurred in 7.6% of cases after the Burch procedure, but only two thirds of these patients required surgical correction. Langer et al. (1988) reported that 13.6% of patients who had undergone a Burch procedure, but no hysterectomy or cul-de-sac obliteration, developed an enterocele 1 to 2 years postoperatively. Alcalay et al. (1995) noted that 26% of patients during a 10- to 20-year follow-up period after Burch colposuspension underwent a rectocele repair and 5% underwent an enterocele repair. Although not all authors agree, performing a Burch colposuspension may increase the risk of developing apical or posterior vaginal prolapse in the future. Whenever possible, a cul-de-sac obliteration in the form of uterosacral plication, Moschcowitz procedure, or McCall culdoplasty should be performed at the time of retropubic colposuspension to prevent enterocele formation, although the true efficacy of this prophylactic maneuver is unknown. Rectocele repair should be done as indicated for symptomatic or large rectoceles; care should be taken to avoid a resulting midvaginal ridge. The postoperative rate of dyspareunia may be 38% when Burch colposuspension and rectocele repair are combined.

Role of Hysterectomy in Treatment of Incontinence

Gynecologists often perform hysterectomies at the time of retropubic or vaginal surgery for SUI. Langer et al. (1988) assessed the effect of concomitant hysterectomy during a Burch colposuspension on the cure rate of SUI. There were 45 patients randomly assigned to receive colposuspension only or colposuspension plus abdominal hysterectomy and cul-de-sac obliteration. Using urodynamics investigations 6 months after surgery, the rate of cure for SUI between the two groups did not differ statistically (95.5% and 95.7% for the no-hysterectomy and hysterectomy groups). This study showed that hysterectomy adds little to the efficacy of Burch colposuspension in curing SUI. Generally, hysterectomies should be performed only for specific uterine pathology or for the treatment of uterovaginal prolapse.

Pregnancy After Retropubic Surgery

Most physicians suggest that the patient finish her childbearing before surgical correction of SUI is attempted. Few data demonstrate the continence status when pregnancy or vaginal delivery occurs after a retropubic repair or sling. Although surgical treatment for stress incontinence generally should be reserved for women who have finished their childbearing, no data convincingly demonstrate that a pregnancy and vaginal delivery would or would not be satisfactory for women after retropubic surgery. Most surgeons prefer not to place polypropylene midurethral slings if the woman desires more pregnancies, although data on this are scarce as well. I believe that an elective cesarean delivery would be an acceptable option for patients who become pregnant after a Burch colposuspension, if desired after careful review of the pertinent risks and benefits.

Suggested Readings

Albo ME, Richter HE, Brubaker L, Norton P, et al. Burch colposuspension versus fascial sling to reduce urinary stress incontinence. *N Engl J Med*. 2007;356:2143.

Alcalay M, Monga A, Stanton SL. Burch colposuspension: a 10-20 year follow up. *Br J Obstet Gynaecol*. 1995;102:740.

Bergman A, Elia G. Three surgical procedures for genuine stress incontinence: five-year follow-up of a prospective randomized study. *Am J Obstet Gynecol*. 1995;173:66.

Bhatia NN, Bergman A. Use of preoperative uroflowmetry and simultaneous urethrocystometry for predicting risk of prolonged postoperative bladder drainage. *Urology* 1986;28:440.

Bidmead J, Cardozo L. Retropubic urethropexy (Burch colposuspension). *Int Urogynecol J*. 2001;12:262.

Black NA, Downs SH. The effectiveness of surgery for stress incontinence in women: a systematic review. *Br J Urol*. 1996;78:497.

Brubaker L, Nygaard I, Richter HE, et al. Two-year outcomes after sacrocolpopexy with and without Burch to prevent stress urinary incontinence. *Obstet Gynecol*. 2008;112:49.

Bump RC, Fantl JA, Hurt WG. Dynamic urethral pressure profilometry pressure transmission ratio determinations after continence surgery: understanding the mechanism of success, failure, and complications. *Obstet Gynecol*. 1988;72:870.

Burch JC. Cooper's ligament urethrovesical suspension for stress incontinence. *Am J Obstet Gynecol*. 1968;100:764.

Burch JC. Urethrovaginal fixation to Cooper's ligament for correction of stress incontinence, cystocele, and prolapse. *Am J Obstet Gynecol*. 1961;81:281.

Cardozo LD, Stanton SL, Williams JE. Detrusor instability following surgery for genuine stress incontinence. *Br J Urol*. 1979;51:204.

Columbo M, Milani R, Vitobello D, et al. A randomized comparison of Burch colposuspension and abdominal paravaginal defect repair for female stress urinary incontinence. *Am J Obstet Gynecol*. 1996;175:78.

Cosson M, Boukerrou M, Narducci F, Occelli B, Querleu D, Crépin G. Long-term results of the Burch procedure combined with abdominal sacrocolpopexy for treatment of vault prolapse. *Int Urogynecol J*. 2003;14:104.

Costantini E, Lazzeri M, Bini V, Del Zingaro M, Zucchi A, Porena M. Burch colposuspension does not provide any additional benefit to pelvic organ prolapse repair in patients with urinary incontinence: a randomized surgical trial. *J Urol*. 2008;180:1007.

Costantini E, Lazzeri M, Bini V, Del Zingaro M, Frumenzio E, Porena M. Pelvic organ prolapse repair with and without concomitant Burch colposuspension in incontinent women: a randomised controlled trial with at least 5-year followup. *Obstet Gynecol Int*. 2012;2012:967923.

Ericksen BC, Hagen B, Eik-Nes SH, et al. Long-term effectiveness of the Burch colposuspension in female urinary stress incontinence. *Acta Obstet Gynecol Scand*. 1990;69:45.

Ferriani RA, Silva de MF, Dias de Moura M, et al. Ureteral blockage as a complication of Burch colposuspension: report of 6 cases. *Gynecol Obstet Invest*. 1990;29:239.

Galloway NTM, Davies N, Stephenson TP. The complications of colposuspension. *Br J Urol*. 1987;60:122.

Herbertsson G, Iosif CS. Surgical results and urodynamic studies 10 years after retropubic colpourethrocystopexy. *Acta Obstet Gynecol Scand*. 1993;72:298.

Hertogs K, Stanton SL. Mechanism of urinary continence after colposuspension: barrier studies. *Br J Obstet Gynaecol*. 1985;92:1184.

Jelovsek JE, Barber MD, Karram MM, Walters MD, Paraiso MF. Randomised trial of laparoscopic Burch colposuspension versus tension-free vaginal tape: long-term follow up. *Br J Obstet Gynaecol*. 2008;115:219.

Karram MM, Bhatia NN. Management of coexistent stress and urge urinary incontinence. *Obstet Gynecol*. 1989;73:4.

Karram M, Maher CF. *Surgical Management of Pelvic Organ Prolapse*. Philadelphia: Saunders; 2013.

Kammerer-Doak DN, Cornella JL, Magrina JF, et al. Osteitis pubis after Marshall-Marchetti-Krantz urethropexy: a pubic osteomyelitis. *Am J Obstet Gynecol*. 1998;179:586.

Kjohede P, Noren B, Ryden G. Prediction of genital prolapse after Burch colposuspension. *Acta Obstet Gynecol Scand.* 1996;75:849.

Kobak WH, Walters MD, Piedmonte MR. Determinants of voiding after three types of incontinence surgery. *Obstet Gynecol.* 2001;97:86.

Kraus SR, Lemack GE, Richter HE, et al; Urinary Incontinence Treatment Network. Changes in urodynamic measures two years after Burch colposuspension or autologous sling surgery. *Urology.* 2011;78:1263.

Kwon CH, Culligan PJ, Koduri S, Goldberg RP, Sand PK. The development of pelvic organ prolapse following isolated Burch retropubic urethropexy. *Int Urogynecol J.* 2003;14:321.

Langer R, Golan A, Ron-El R, et al. Colposuspension for urinary stress incontinence in premenopausal and postmenopausal women. *Surg Gynecol Obstet.* 1990;171:13.

Langer R, Ron-El R, Neuman N, et al. The value of simultaneous hysterectomy during Burch colposuspension for urinary stress incontinence. *Obstet Gynecol.* 1988;72:866.

Lapitan MC, Cody JD, Grant A. Open retropubic colposuspension for urinary incontinence in women. *Cochrane Database Syst Rev.* 2009;(2):CD002912. [Update in *Cochrane Database Syst Rev.* 2009; (4):CD002912.]

Laursen H, Farlie R, Rasmussen KL, et al. Colposuspension Burch: an 18 year follow-up study. *Neurourol Urodyn.* 1994;13:445.

Lind LR, Gunn GC, Mattox TF, Stanford EJ. Mini-incision Burch urethropexy: a less invasive method to accomplish a time-tested procedure for treatment of genuine stress incontinence. *Int Urogynecol J.* 2004;15:20.

Mainprize TC, Drutz HP. The Marshall-Marchetti-Krantz procedure: a critical review. *Obstet Gynecol Surv.* 1988;43:724.

Marshall VF, Marchetti AA, Krantz KE. The correction of stress incontinence by simple vesicourethral suspension. *Surg Gynecol Obstet.* 1949;88:509.

Meltomaa SS, Haarala MA, Taalikka MO, Kiiholma PJ, Alanen A, Makinen JI. Outcome of Burch retropubic urethropexy and the effect of concomitant abdominal hysterectomy: a prospective long-term follow-up study. *Int Urogynecol J.* 2001;12:3.

Moon YJ, Jeon MJ, Kim SK, Bai SW. Comparison of Burch colposuspension and transobturator tape when combined with abdominal sacrocolpopexy. *Int J Gynaecol Obstet.* 2011;112:122.

Novara G, Artibani W, Barber MD, et al. Updated systematic review and meta-analysis of the comparative data on colposuspensions, pubovaginal slings, and midurethral tapes in the surgical treatment of female stress urinary incontinence. *Eur Urol.* 2010;58:218.

Richardson AC, Edmonds PB, Williams NL. Treatment of stress urinary incontinence due to paravaginal fascial defect. *Obstet Gynecol.* 1981;57:357.

Richter HE, Diokno A, Kenton K, et al; Urinary Incontinence Treatment Network. Predictors of treatment failure 24 months after surgery for stress urinary incontinence. *J Urol.* 2008;179:1024.

Rosenthal RE, Spickard WA, Markham RD, et al. Osteomyelitis of the symphysis pubis: a separate disease from osteitis pubis. *J Bone Joint Surg Am.* 1982;64:123.

Sand PK, Bowen LW, Ostergard DR, et al. Hysterectomy and prior surgery as risk factors for failed retropubic cystourethropexy. *J Reprod Med.* 1988;33:171.

Sand PK, Bowen LW, Panganiban R, et al. The low pressure urethra as a factor in failed retropubic urethropexy. *Obstet Gynecol.* 1987;69:399.

Shull BL. How I do the abdominal paravaginal repair. *J Pelvic Surg.* 1995;1:43.

Shull BL, Baden WF. A six-year experience with paravaginal defect repair for stress urinary incontinence. *Am J Obstet Gynecol.* 1989;160:1432.

Stanton SL, Cardozo L, Williams JE, et al. Clinical and urodynamic features of failed incontinence surgery in the female. *Obstet Gynecol.* 1978;51:515.

Steel SA, Cox C, Stanton SL. Long-term follow-up of detrusor instability following the colposuspension operation. *Br J Urol.* 1986;58:138.

Tanagho EA. Colpocystourethropexy: the way we do it. *J Urol.* 1976;116:751.

Turner-Warwick R. Turner-Warwick vagino-obturator shelf urethral repositioning procedure. In: Debruyne FMJ, van Kerrebroeck EVA, eds. *Practical Aspects of Urinary Incontinence.* Dordrecht, The Netherlands: Martinus Nijhoff; 1986.

Turner-Warwick RT. The pathogenesis and treatment of osteitis pubis. *Br J Urol.* 1960;32:464.

Wang AC, Chen M. Comparison of tension-free vaginal taping versus modified Burch colposuspension on urethral obstruction: a randomized controlled trial. *Neurourol Urodyn.* 2003;22:185.

Ward K, Hilton P. Prospective multicentre randomized trial of tension-free vaginal tape and colposuspension as primary treatment for stress incontinence. *BMJ* 2002;325:1.

Ward K, Hilton P. A prospective multicenter randomized trial of tension-free vaginal tape and colposuspension for primary urodynamic stress incontinence: two-year follow-up. *Am J Obstet Gynecol.* 2004;190:324.

Weber AM, Walters MD, Piedmonte MR. Sexual function and vaginal anatomy in women before and after surgery for pelvic organ prolapse and urinary incontinence. *Am J Obstet Gynecol* 2000;182:1610.

Webster GD, Kreder KJ. Voiding dysfunction following cystourethropexy: its evaluation and management. *J Urol.* 1990;144:670.

Wiskind AK, Creighton SM, Stanton SL. The incidence of genital prolapse after the Burch colposuspension. *Am J Obstet Gynecol.* 1992;167:399.

Biologic Bladder Neck Pubovaginal Slings

Mickey Karram, M.D.
Dani Zoorob, M.D.
W. Stuart Reynolds, M.D.
Melissa R. Kaufman, M.D.
Roger Dmochowski, M.D.

  Videos

5-1 Rectus Fascia Pubovaginal Sling Procedure

5-2 Urethral Reconstruction with Martius Fat Pad Transposition and Cadaveric Fascia Lata Pubovaginal Sling

Introduction

The concept of using a patient's own tissue as a "sling" to support the urethra dates back to the beginning of the 20th century; however, it was not until the last quarter of the 20th century that the procedure gained widespread popularity and evolved into its current state. Initially, the procedure was described as using a strip of mobilized abdominal muscle (either rectus or pyramidalis). One end of the strip was freed from its attachment, passed under the bladder neck, and then reaffixed to the abdominal muscle wall, forming a "U"-shaped sling of muscle around the bladder outlet. Subsequently, overlying abdominal fascia was also included in the sling and eventually replaced the muscle altogether. The final innovation involved using an isolated strip of fascia suspended by free sutures that were tied to the abdominal wall directly or on top of the abdominal rectus sheath.

Despite originating as an autologous procedure, many different types of materials have been used as sling substitutions, including various sources of autologous tissue, allograft tissue, xenograft tissue, and synthetic material. Almost all these substitutions have been made in an attempt to limit patient morbidity by alleviating the additional morbidity created by the harvesting of the sling material. Nevertheless, the most popular pubovaginal sling still uses autologous rectus abdominis fascia. Regardless of the material used, the pubovaginal sling is meant to be placed at the junction of the proximal urethra and bladder neck for purposes of supporting the urethra, as well as augmenting intraurethral pressure and deficient proximal sphincteric function.

Continence is achieved either by providing a direct compressive force on the urethra/bladder outlet or by reestablishing a reinforcing platform or hammock against which the urethra is compressed during transmission of increased abdominal pressure. The sling is suspended with free sutures on each end that either are attached directly to the abdominal wall musculature or more commonly are tied to each other on the anterior surface of the abdominal wall. The long-term success of the procedure relies not on the integrity of the suspensory sutures, but rather on the healing and fibrotic process involving the sling, which occurs primarily where the sling passes through the endopelvic fascia.

Indications

The pubovaginal sling is a treatment option for stress urinary incontinence (SUI). Although pioneered as a surgical option for intrinsic sphincter deficiency, the indications have been broadened to encompass all types of SUI. Because of its reliable results and durable outcomes, it is considered to be one of the main standards of treatment of SUI and has been used extensively as a primary therapy of SUI both for intrinsic sphincter deficiency and for urethral hypermobility, as a salvage procedure for recurrent SUI, as an adjunct for urethral and bladder reconstruction, and even as a way to "close" the urethra functionally to abandon urethral access to the bladder altogether. In our opinion, other indications are in patients with SUI who decline to have a synthetic material implanted because of concerns related to the long-term presence of synthetic mesh. Also, women who have recurrent incontinence after a synthetic sling or have had a complication after a synthetic sling such as a vaginal erosion may be good candidates for a biologic sling. Finally, we prefer to use a biologic sling in patients who have undergone radiation or who have had urethral injuries and patients who are undergoing either simultaneous or prior urethrovaginal fistula or diverticulum repair.

Sling Materials

Several different types of materials have been tried and investigated for use as a pubovaginal sling. The two most common autologous tissues are rectus abdominis fascia and fascia lata. Both have been extensively studied and have proven to be efficacious and reliable. Of the two, most surgeons prefer rectus abdominis fascia as an autologous material because it is easier and quicker to harvest.

Other biologic materials that have been used include allogeneic (i.e., cadaveric) and xenogeneic tissues. Cadaveric fascia lata and cadaveric dermis provide reasonable efficacy; however, durability of results remains an issue because high failure rates have been reported in some studies. Bovine and porcine dermis and porcine small intestine submucosa have also demonstrated acceptable efficacy for SUI, but durability again remains a concern.

Synthetic graft materials of various designs and substances have also been used as sling material. As with other types of synthetic graft materials, monofilament, large-pore weave grafts (type 1 mesh) are recommended for implantation in the vagina. Good efficacy can be achieved with synthetic mesh; however, synthetic mesh also poses risks of serious complications, including infection, vaginal extrusion, and genitourinary erosion, and is currently not recommended for use underneath the proximal urethra or bladder neck.

Technique for Harvest of Rectus Fascia and Placement of Pubovaginal Sling

1. *Preoperative considerations.* Pubovaginal sling procedures are generally performed under general anesthesia, but spinal or epidural anesthesia is also possible. Full patient paralysis is not warranted but may facilitate rectus fascia closure after fascial harvest. Perioperative antibiotics are usually administered with appropriate skin and vaginal floral coverage (e.g., a cephalosporin or fluoroquinolone). (Antibiotic prophylaxis has now become a mandated quality of care measure in the United States.)

2. *Positioning.* The patient is placed in the low lithotomy position with legs in stirrups, and the abdomen and perineum are sterilely prepared and draped to provide access to the vagina and the lower abdomen. The bladder is drained with a Foley catheter. A weighted vaginal speculum is placed, and either lateral labial retraction sutures are placed or a self-retaining retractor system is employed to facilitate vaginal exposure.

3. *Abdominal incision.* An 8- to 10-cm Pfannenstiel incision is made (approximately 3 to 5 cm above the pubic bone), and the dissection is carried down to the level of the rectus fascia with a combination of electrocautery and blunt dissection, sweeping the fat and subcutaneous tissue clear of the rectus abdominus fascia (Figure 5-1).

4. *Fascial harvest.* Harvest of the rectus abdominis fascia can be carried out in a transverse or vertical orientation. Typically, a fascial segment measuring at least 8 cm in length and 1.5 to 2 cm in width is harvested. The fascial segment to be resected is delineated with a surgical marking pen or electrocautery and incised sharply with a scalpel, scissors, or electrocautery along the drawn lines. Although virgin fascia is preferred, fibrotic rectus fascia can also be used. If resecting the fascia close and parallel to the symphysis pubis, it is advisable to leave at least 2 to 3 cm of fascia attached to the bone to facilitate closure and approximation to the superior fascial edge. Use of small Army-Navy retractors permits aggressive retraction of skin edges, allowing access through a smaller skin incision (Figure 5-2).

5. *Fascial defect closure.* The fascial defect is closed using a heavy gauge (No. 1 or 0), delayed absorbable suture in a running fashion. Mobilization of the rectus abdominis fascial edges may be required to ensure appropriate tension-free approximation. It is important to ensure adequate anesthesia with muscular relaxation or paralysis when the closure is being done.

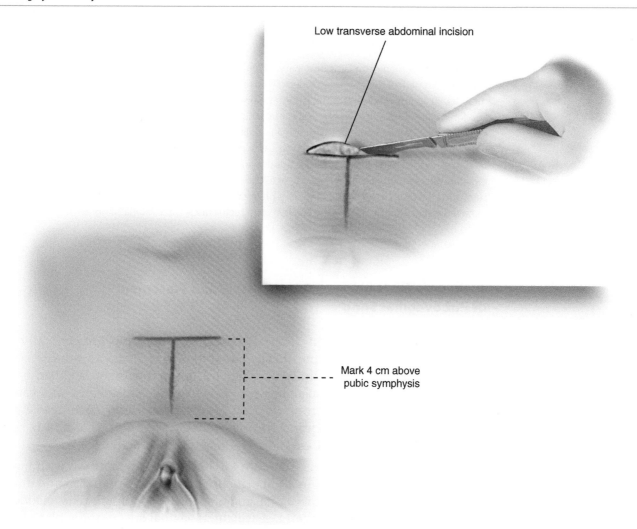

Low transverse abdominal incision

Mark 4 cm above
pubic symphysis

Figure 5-1 The location of the skin incision is delineated before initiating the procedure. The incision should measure about 8 to 10 cm and be located about 4 cm above the symphysis pubis. A vertical incision is also feasible, although often less esthetic.

6. *Preparation of fascia.* To prepare the fascial sling for use, a No. 1 permanent (e.g., polypropylene) suture is affixed to each end using a figure-of-eight stitch to secure the suture to the sling. Defatting of the sling may be done if necessary (Figure 5-3).

7. *Vaginal dissection.* Vaginal dissection proceeds with a midline or inverted "U" incision. Injectable-grade saline or local analgesic, such as 1% lidocaine, may be used to hydrodissect the subepithelial tissues. Vaginal flaps are created with sufficient mobility to ensure tension-free closure over the sling. Dissection is carried laterally and anteriorly until the endopelvic fascia is encountered. The endopelvic fascia is incised and dissected from the posterior surface of the pubis to allow entrance into the retropubic space. This dissection sometimes can be done bluntly but often, especially in recurrent cases, requires sharp dissection with Mayo scissors (Figure 5-4).

8. *Passing retropubic needles or clamp.* Stamey needles or long clamps are passed through the retropubic space from the open abdominal wound immediately posterior to the pubic bone, approximately 4 cm apart. Distal control of the needles is maintained by direct finger guidance through the vaginal incision, and the tip of the needle is advanced adjacent to the

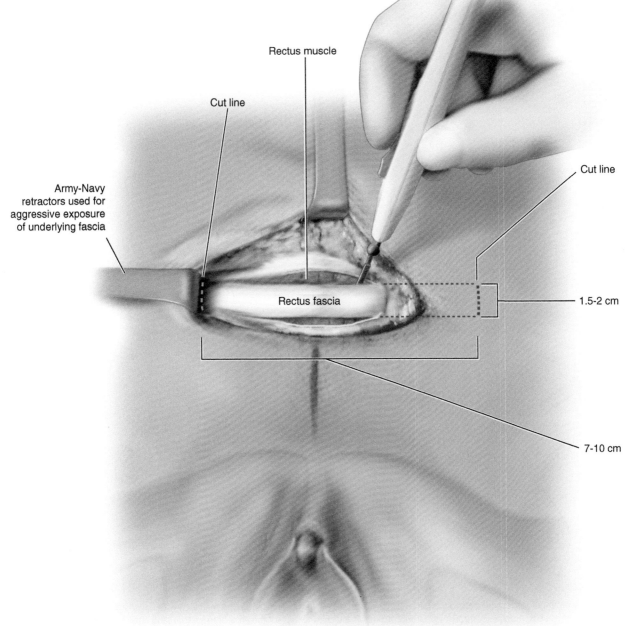

Rectus muscle

Cut line

Cut line

Army-Navy
retractors used for
aggressive exposure
of underlying fascia

Rectus fascia

1.5-2 cm

7-10 cm

Figure 5-2 Fascial strip resection. After deciding on the optimal location for excision, the area is marked with electrocautery or a surgical marking pen. Strip resection is accomplished using a scalpel or electrocautery. The strip should measure 8 to 10 cm and be 1 to 2 cm wide. When attempting to use a small skin incision, Army-Navy retractors may be helpful in enhancing exposure.

posterior surface of the pubic bone to avoid inadvertent bladder injury. Proper bladder drainage must be ensured to minimize injury to the bladder, which may be closely adherent to the pubis, especially if a prior retropubic procedure, as in the case presented, has been performed (Figure 5-5).

9. *Cystoscopy*. Careful cystoscopic examination of the bladder after passing the needles is mandatory to rule out inadvertent bladder injury. Injuries to the bladder typically occur at the 1 o'clock and 11 o'clock positions. The bladder must be completely filled to expand any mucosal redundancy. Movement

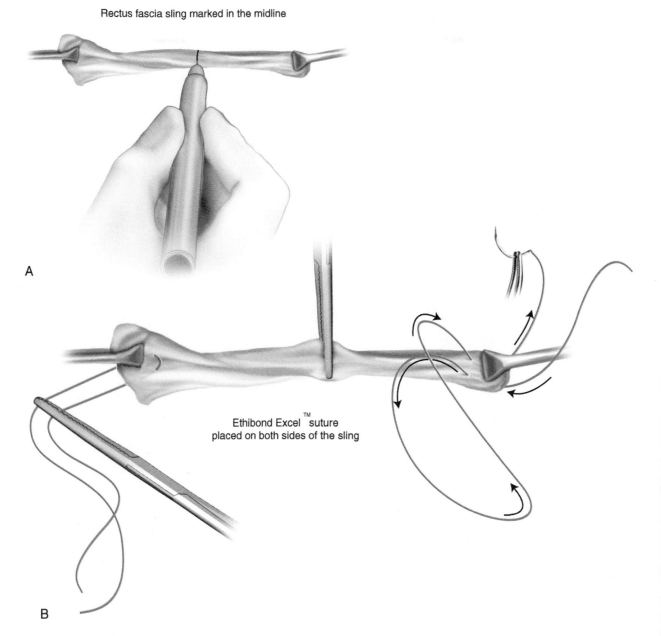

Rectus fascia sling marked in the midline

A

Ethibond Excel ™ suture
placed on both sides of the sling

B

Figure 5-3 Attachment of suspensory arms to the fascial sling. **A,** The midline of the fascial sling is demarcated with a marking pen, and the sling is gently grasped with a hemostat. **B,** A polyester suture (e.g., Ethibond Excel) is attached to each of the ends of the fascial sling after stripping the sling of any adipose tissue attached to it. The surgeon ensures that the initial entry and exit points of the polyester sutures are on the same side of the strip originally abutting the rectus muscles.

of the needles or clamps can help to localize their position relative to the bladder wall.

10. *Deploying.* To deploy the sling, the free ends of the sutures affixed to the sling are threaded into the ends of the Stamey needles or grasped with the clamp, and each suture is pulled up to the anterior abdominal wall through the retropubic space. Care is taken to maintain the orientation of the sling so that it is centered and flat at the bladder neck area (Figure 5-6).

11. Some surgeons prefer to fix the sling in the midline to the underlying periurethral tissue with numerous delayed absorbable sutures. However, we prefer to leave the sling unattached to the underlying urethra and bladder neck.

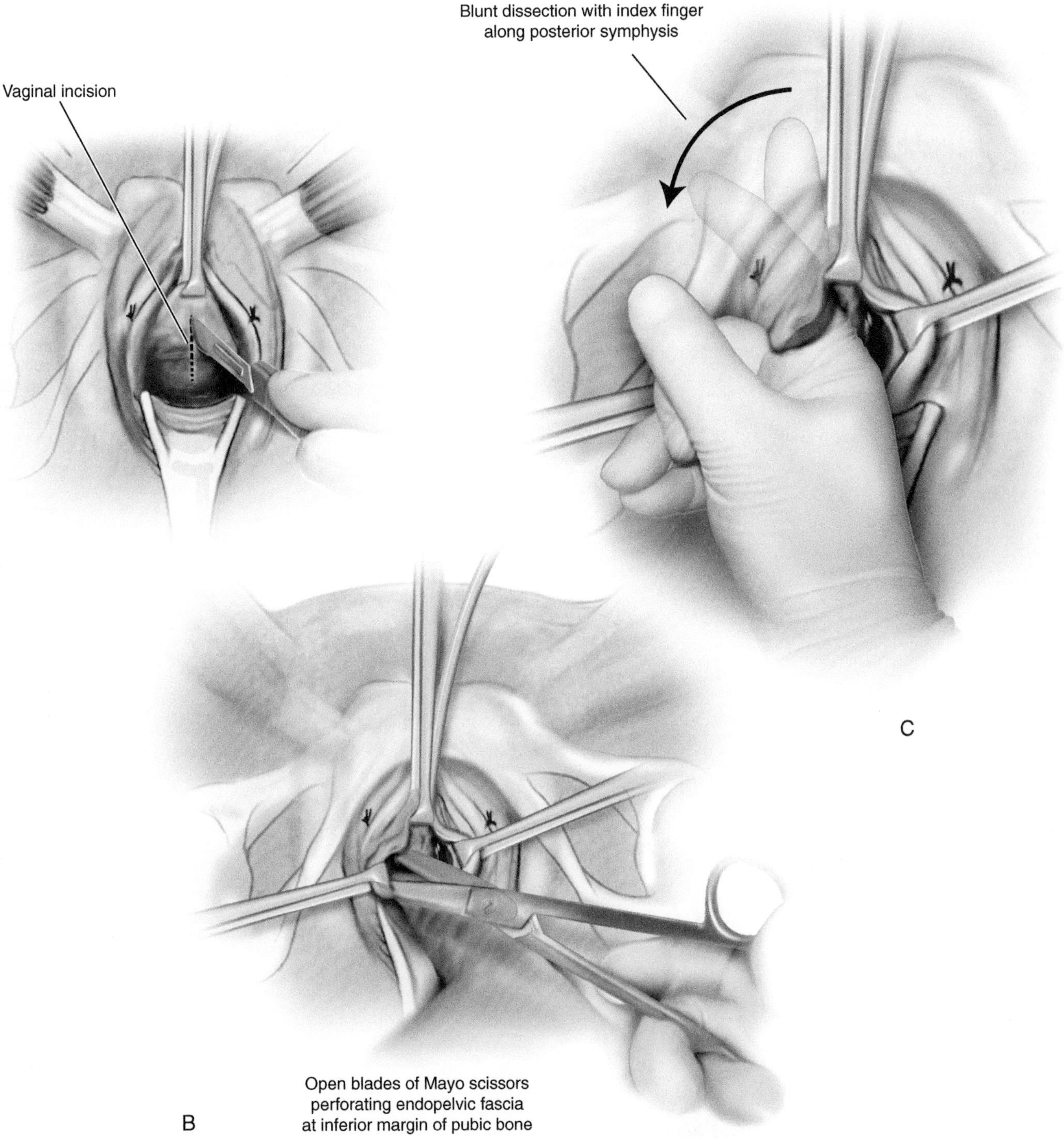

Blunt dissection with index finger
along posterior symphysis

Vaginal incision

C

Open blades of Mayo scissors
perforating endopelvic fascia
B   at inferior margin of pubic bone

Figure 5-4 Vaginal dissection. **A,** A vertical or inverted "U"–shaped incision is used on the vaginal mucosa overlying the midurethra and bladder. **B,** Careful dissection is carried out to the pubic rami bilaterally until the urogenital diaphragm is identified. The urogenital diaphragm is sharply penetrated with the help of Mayo scissors. **C,** To develop the space, the opening created should be digitally enlarged by sweeping the index finger against the arch of the symphysis pubis. The same procedure is repeated on the opposite side.

12. *Tensioning of the sling.* Various techniques for tensioning of the sling are applicable. To ensure adequate "looseness," we prefer to tie the sutures across the midline while holding a right-angled clamp between the sling material and the posterior urethral surface. Tensioning of the sling may also be accomplished by direct vision of proximal/bladder neck coaptation with rigid cystoscopy while gently pulling up on the free ends of the sling sutures.

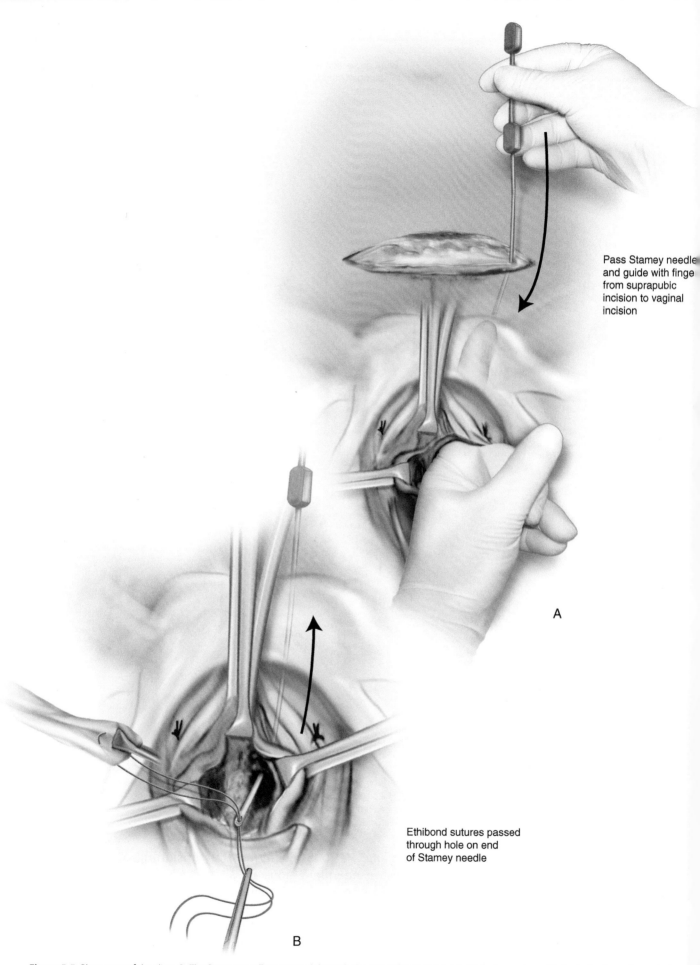

Pass Stamey needle and guide with finge from suprapubic incision to vaginal incision

A

Ethibond sutures passed through hole on end of Stamey needle

B

Figure 5-5 Placement of the sling. **A,** The Stamey needle is inserted through the rectus fascia and guided into the vagina with the index finger in contact with the tip of the needle. **B,** Both ends of the polyester suture are threaded into the eye of the Stamey needle, and the needle is pulled back up through the retropubic space and delivered abdominally at the level of the fascia.

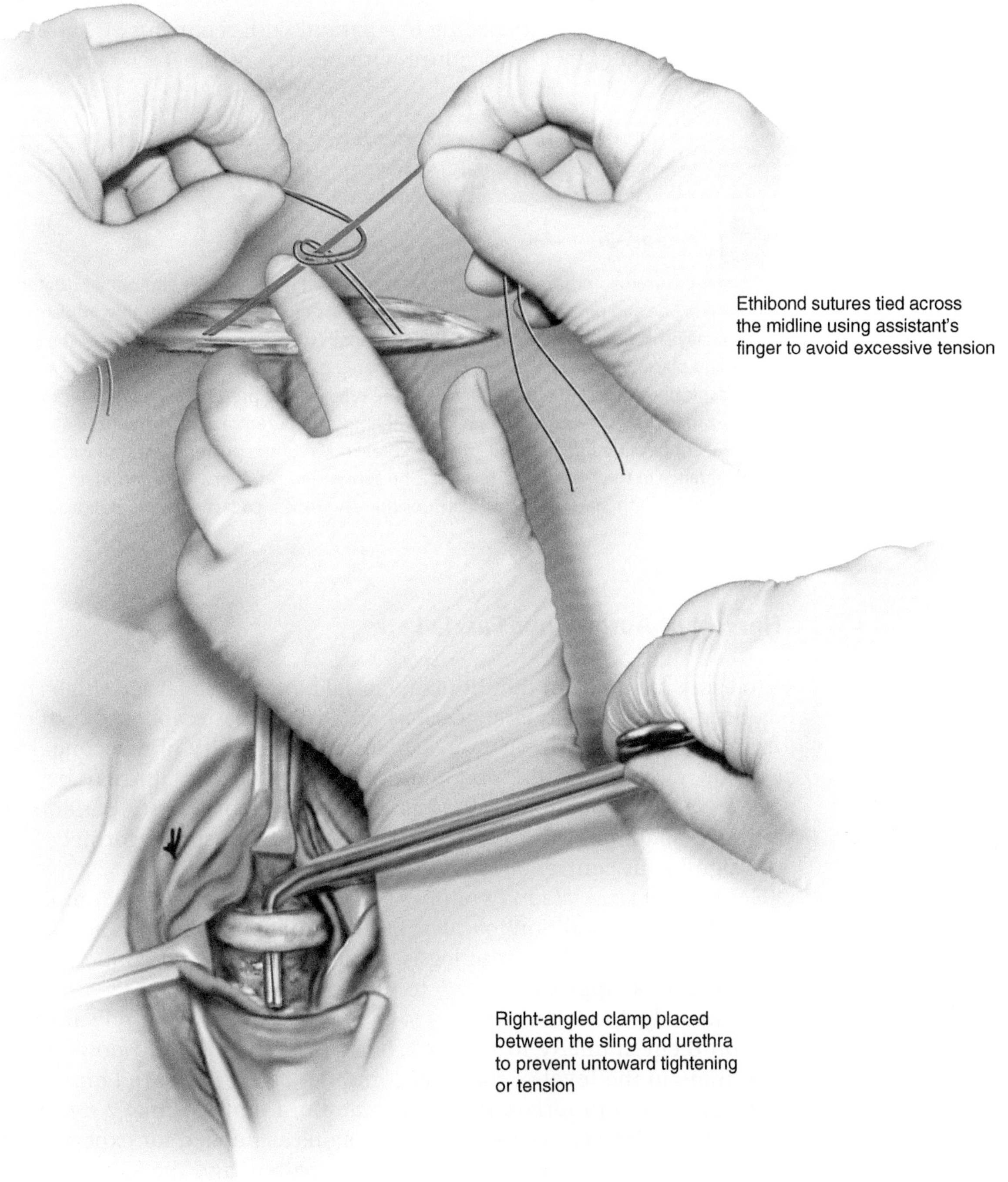

Ethibond sutures tied across the midline using assistant's finger to avoid excessive tension

Right-angled clamp placed between the sling and urethra to prevent untoward tightening or tension

Figure 5-6 Tensioning of the sling. Sling tensioning is accomplished by tying the suspensory sutures abdominally above the fascial closure line. The sutures are tied across the assistant's index finger to avoid excessive tensioning. This is done concurrently with a right-angled clamp being placed between the pubovaginal sling and the vagina.

13. The abdominal skin incision is closed with 3-0 and 4-0 absorbable sutures. The vaginal mucosa is closed with 3-0 absorbable sutures. We prefer to close the vagina after the tensioning procedure has been completed, whereas some surgeons complete this step before the tensioning.

14. A bladder catheter is left indwelling, and vaginal gauze packing is placed. The catheter and vaginal packing may be removed after 24 hours. If the patient is unable to void, she is taught intermittent self-catheterization or an indwelling Foley catheter is left in place for 1 week.

See **Video 5-1** for demonstration of the harvest of the rectus fascia and placement of a pubovaginal sling in a patient with recurrent SUI after a tension-free vaginal tape (TVT) procedure with erosion of the TVT tape.

Case 2: Placement of a Biologic Pubovaginal Sling in a Patient with Complete Loss of Posterior Urethra

(Video 5-2)

A 35-year-old woman presents with urinary leakage that is continuous and not associated with movement. She had previously been given a diagnosis of an ectopic ureter that implanted into a congenitally short urethra. She had undergone repairs including reimplantation of the ectopic ureter and placement of a cadaveric fascia lata sling. A congenital remnant, noted as a blind pouch cystoscopically, was left in place attached to the urethra. She presented 2 years after this repair, and pelvic examination showed complete loss of the posterior urethra. It was theorized at the time that this remnant became infected and created a breakdown of the posterior urethra with complete disappearance of the cadaveric fascia lata. She subsequently underwent a complete urethral reconstruction with Martius fat pad transposition and repeat cadaveric fascia pubovaginal sling.

Harvest of Autologous Fascia Lata

Autologous tissue from the iliotibial fascial band of the lateral thigh (fascia lata) has been used with great success as an alternative to abdominal rectus fascia for a pubovaginal sling. Although incurring morbidity of a secondary incision at a site remote from the abdomen, harvesting fascia lata may be suitable in patients in whom abdominal fascia may be of poor quality patients in whom extensive abdominal procedures have been previously performed, or patients with significant central obesity or a large pannus.

Harvest of fascia lata may require separate positioning, skin preparation, and sterile draping in addition to that for the vaginal procedure. To access the lateral aspect of the distal thigh, the leg is medially rotated and adducted. Two transverse incisions, approximately 5 to 6 cm in length, are made: a distal incision approximately 4 to 6 cm superior to the lateral femoral condyle and a proximal incision 8 cm cranially to the first. The incision is carried down through the fatty tissue to the level of the fascia, and the fascia is cleared either sharply or bluntly for an appropriate distance to attain a graft 8 cm × 2 cm in size. The fascial strip is harvested, using both incisions as needed for exposure. Once the graft is removed, the fascial defect is not repaired, and the subcutaneous tissue and skin are closed in multiple layers with absorbable suture. A Penrose drain can be secured in place through a separate stab incision and may be removed after 24 hours. Alternatively, a dedicated fascial stripper may be used for graft harvest when a full strip of fascia is desired.

Outcomes

The literature shows that pubovaginal slings are highly effective with success rates of 50% to 75% when followed for 10 years (Norton and Brubaker 2006). In 2011, Blaivas and Chaikin reported 4-year follow-up with improvement or cure in 100% of patients with uncomplicated SUI and 93% in the more complicated cases. These authors reported that most failures were due to urge incontinence and occurred within the first 6 months postoperatively; 3% of patients with urge incontinence were believed to have developed de novo urge incontinence.

Other studies reported development of de novo urgency and storage symptoms in 23% of patients with 11% of patients reporting voiding dysfunction and 7.8% requiring long-term self-catheterization (Norton and Brubaker 2006). The few randomized controlled trials comparing pubovaginal slings with TVT have had flawed methodology, and their outcomes are questionable (Novara et al., 2010). Basok et al. (2008) showed an increased rate of de novo urgency in the pubovaginal sling group compared with intravaginal slingplasty, whereas Sharifiaghdas and Mortazavi (2008) noted equal efficacy when they retrospectively compared an autologous pubovaginal sling to a retropubic synthetic midurethral sling. The most scientifically valid randomized controlled trial was by Arunkalaivanan in 2003, and it showed equal subjective cure rates and complication rates when a biologic pubovaginal sling was compared with TVT. In this study, the pubovaginal sling was of a porcine origin. When comparing autologous versus allograft slings, Flynn and Yap (2002) showed equal effectiveness in control of SUI over 2 years with reduced postoperative discomfort in the allograft group. Both groups had recurrent SUI develop in up to 10% of patients. Autologous pubovaginal slings were compared with Burch colposuspension in a multicenter randomized controlled trial (SISTEr Trial), noting superiority of fascial slings in controlling incontinence, despite an increased morbidity profile (Albo et al., 2007). In a meta-analysis in 2010, pubovaginal and midurethral synthetic slings were compared; equal subjective cure rates and equal overall effectiveness were reported (Novara et al., 2010).

Complications

Needle Bladder Injuries

If inadvertent bladder injury occurs during retropubic passage of the Stamey needle and is recognized in a timely manner on cystoscopy, the needle can simply be withdrawn and repassed through the retropubic space, and the procedure can be continued as planned. An unrecognized bladder injury can result in serious complications related to foreign body reactions in the bladder, including suture and sling erosion into the bladder, stone formation, and voiding dysfunction.

Pelvic Visceral Injuries and Blood Loss

Pelvic visceral injuries and pelvic hematomas are rare and can be avoided or minimized by adequate dissection of the endopelvic fascia and retropubic space and careful needle passage in close proximity to the posterior surface of the pubic bone with distal needle control with the surgeon's finger. If an inadvertent cystotomy or urethrotomy were to occur, the injury should be appropriately repaired. In contrast to synthetic sling placement, which would commonly require aborting the procedure, a biologic sling could still be placed after concurrent intraoperative repair of the injury.

Miscellaneous Surgical Complications

Superficial wound infection, subcutaneous seromas, and abdominal fascial hernias are uncommon. In obese patients, the use of a subcutaneous drain may be required to prevent fluid loculations. Sling erosions with autologous tissue are exceedingly rare.

Voiding Dysfunction

Transient urinary retention may occur in 20% of patients and requires intermittent self-catheterization until resolution (typically 2 to 4 weeks). Prolonged (persisting >4 to 6 weeks) postoperative voiding dysfunction, including de novo urgency, urgency incontinence, or obstructive symptoms, may occur to some degree in 25% of patients. Less than 3% of women require subsequent urethrolysis for treatment of prolonged retention or obstructive voiding symptoms. Some surgeons routinely teach patients intermittent self-catheterization in the preoperative period to facilitate its use, if necessary, postoperatively.

Surgical Tips

1. Because substantial bleeding can occur during vaginal dissection, harvesting the autologous fascia and preparing the sling by affixing sutures should be performed first, before vaginal dissection, so that the sling may be inserted and deployed in a timely manner and blood loss can be minimized. Retropubic bleeding occurring during dissection almost always resolves with sling placement, and time should not be spent on prolonged attempts at hemostasis.

2. When performing an autologous pubovaginal sling procedure in the setting of urethral reconstruction (e.g., urethrovaginal fistula or diverticulum resection) or as tissue interposition, harvesting fascia and preparing and deploying the sling with passage of the retropubic sutures, but not tensioning, should be performed before the delicate urethral reconstruction. When the reconstruction is finished, the sling can be affixed in the appropriate location and tensioned. Damage to the reconstruction can occur through traction or direct injury if the sling is deployed after reconstruction.

3. Surface orientation of the autologous sling material during placement of the graft does not matter; by convention, the body "side" or underside of the graft is placed on the body "side" of the patient.

4. For most women, sling tensioning can be accomplished with the "two finger" distance over the fascia. However, in women who have had multiple procedures and have a nonmobile urethra, the sling tension should be more significant, using a one-fingerbreadth knot with concomitant cystoscopic evidence of an impression ("lip or ledge") being created on the ventrum of the urethra.

Conclusion

Pubovaginal slings using a biologic sling material (whether autologous, allograft, or xenograft) can be employed successfully to manage primary or recurrent SUI.

Suggested Readings

Albo ME, Richter HE, Brubaker L, et al. Randomized trial of porcine dermal sling (Pelvicol implant) vs. tension-free vaginal tape (TVT) in the surgical treatment of stress incontinence: a questionnaire-based study. *Int Urogynecol J Pelvic Floor Dysfunct.* 2003;14:17-23.

Albo ME, Richter HE, Brubaker L, et al. Burch colposuspension versus fascial sling to reduce urinary stress incontinence. *N Engl J Med.* 2007;356:2143-2155.

Arunkalaivanan AS, Barrington JW. Randomized trial of porcine dermal sling (Pelvicol implant) vs tension-free vaginal tape (TVT) in the surgical treatment of stress; a questionnaire-based study. *Int Urogynecol J Pelvic Floor Dysfunct.* 2003;14(1):17.

Basok EK, Yildirim A, Atsu N, Basaran A, Tokuc R. Cadaveric fascia lata versus intravaginal slingplasty for the pubovaginal sling: surgical outcome, overall success and patient satisfaction rates. *Urol Int.* 2008;80:46-51.

Blaivas JG, Chaikin DC. Pubovaginal fascial sling for the treatment of all types of stress urinary incontinence: surgical technique and long-term outcome. *Urol Clin North Am.* 2011;38:7-15.

Blaivas JG, Olsson CA. Stress incontinence: classification and surgical approach. *J Urol.* 1988;139: 727-731.

Chaikin DC, Rosenthal J, Blaivas JG. Pubovaginal fascial sling for all types of stress urinary incontinence: long-term analysis. *J Urol.* 1998;160:1312-1316.

Dmochowski RR, Blaivas JM, Gormley EA, et al. Update of AUA guideline on the surgical management of female stress urinary incontinence. *J Urol.* 2010;183:1906-1914.

Flynn BJ, Yap WT. Pubovaginal sling using autograft fascia for all types of stress urinary incontinence: 2-year minimum followup. *J Urol.* 2002;167(2 Pt 1):608-612.

Gomelsky A, Dmochowski RR. Bladder neck pubovaginal slings. *Expert Rev Med Devices.* 2005; 2:327-340.

Groutz A, Blaivas JG, Hyman MJ, Chaikin DC. Pubovaginal sling surgery for simple stress urinary incontinence: analysis by an outcome score. *J Urol.* 2001;165:1597-1600.

McGuire EJ, Lytton B. Pubovaginal sling procedure for stress incontinence. 1978. *J Urol.* 2002;167:1120-1123; discussion 1124.

Morgan TO Jr, Westney OL, McGuire EJ. Pubovaginal sling: 4-year outcome analysis and quality of life assessment. *J Urol.* 2000;163:1845-1848.

Norton P, Brubaker L. Urinary incontinence in women. *Lancet.* 2006;367:57-67.

Novara G, Artibani W, Barber MD, et al. Updated systematic review and meta-analysis of the comparative data on colposuspensions, pubovaginal slings, and midurethral tapes in the surgical treatment of female stress urinary incontinence. *Eur Urol.* 2010;58:218-238.

Sharifiaghdas F, Mortazavi N. Tension-free vaginal tape and autologous rectus fascia pubovaginal sling for the treatment of urinary stress incontinence: a medium-term follow-up. *Med Princ Pract.* 2008;17:209-214.

Smith ARB, Dmochowski R, Hilton P, et al; Committee 14. Surgery for urinary incontinence in women. In: Abrams P, Cardozo L, Khoury S, Wein A, eds. *Incontinence: 4th International Consultation on Incontinence.* Paris: Health Publication Ltd; 2009:1191-1272.

Tcherniakovsky M, Fernandes CE, Bezerra CA, et al. Comparative results of two techniques to treat stress urinary incontinence: synthetic transobturator and aponeurotic slings. *Intern Urogynecol J.* 2009;20:961-966.

Wilson WJ, Winters JC. Is there still a place for the pubovaginal sling at the bladder neck in the era of the midurethral sling? *Curr Urol Rep.* 2005;6:335-339.

Zyczynski H, Diokno AC, Tennstedt S, et al; Urinary Incontinence Treatment Network. Burch colposuspension versus fascial sling to reduce urinary stress incontinence. *N Engl J Med.* 2007;356:2143-2155.

Retropubic Synthetic Midurethral Slings

Mickey Karram, M.D.
Dani Zoorob, M.D.
W. Stuart Reynolds, M.D.
Melissa R. Kaufman, M.D.
Roger Dmochowski, M.D.

6

 Videos

6-1 Traditional Tension-Free Vaginal Tape Procedure

6-2 Tension-Free Vaginal Tape EXACT Procedure

6-3 SPARC Procedure

Introduction

Synthetic midurethral slings (MUS) have become the most popular incontinence procedures performed in the 21st century. No other innovation for the treatment of stress urinary incontinence (SUI) has had more appeal to surgeons and patients. These procedures are minimally invasive, have a high efficacy rate with very low morbidity, and have a quick recovery period. This chapter and the following two chapters discuss the currently available synthetic MUS on the market.

Retropubic MUS were developed in the mid-1990s in an attempt to create a minimally invasive surgical treatment for SUI. Up until this time incontinence procedures were aimed at suspending or supporting the proximal urethra and bladder neck. In 1995, Ulmsten and Petros described a rationale for a more distally placed suburethral sling based on concepts they termed the "integral theory." This theory was based on the presumption that the pubourethral ligaments support the midurethra and attach to the pubic bones, acting as a backboard for the midurethra. This backboard allows the compression of the midurethra against it when intraabdominal pressure increases and maintains continence. The concept states that the absence of the backboard support causes a loss of this watertight seal, and SUI develops. By passing a strip of supportive material (loosely woven polypropylene) under the midurethra in women with SUI, this "backboard" action could theoretically be replicated. The strip of polypropylene was to be left loose or "tension-less," and direct compression of the urethra was avoided. In its earliest configuration, placement of the MUS was achieved through an anterior vaginal wall dissection at the level of the midurethra. Placement of the sling material was accomplished by passage of the arms of the tape in a retropubic fashion through the anterior abdominal wall with the aid of specially designed trocars.

Figure 6-1 A, Tension-free vaginal tape instrumentation, including *(clockwise from top)* a Foley catheter guide, a needle introducer/handle, and specially designed needles attached to a synthetic suburethral sling tape. **B,** Needles have been attached to the handle. A hemostat has been placed on the overlapping plastic sheath.

(From Baggish MS, Karram MM, eds. Atlas of Pelvic Anatomy and Gynecology Surgery, *ed 3. St. Louis: Saunders; 2011.)*

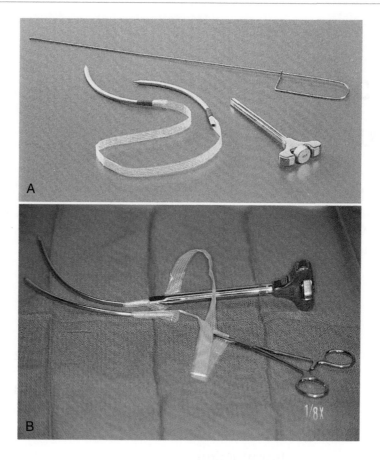

Table 6–1 Commercially available retropubic midurethral sling kits

Sling	Manufacturer	Trocar Passage
TVT	Ethicon, Somerville, NJ	Bottom-up
SPARC Sling System	American Medical Systems, Minnetonka, MN	Top-down
LYNX Suprapubic MUS System	Boston Scientific, Natick, MA	Top-down
Advantage Fit System	Boston Scientific	Bottom-up
Align Retropubic	Band Medical, Covington, GA	Bottom-up and top-down

The first commercially available retropubic MUS was the tension-free vaginal tape (Gynecare, Somerville, NJ) (Figure 6-1), which consisted of a narrow polypropylene mesh strip with two specially designed trocars that were inserted through a small vaginal incision and passed through the retropubic space to an exit point in the suprapubic area of the anterior abdominal wall. Passage of the trocars from the vaginal incision to the anterior abdominal wall has been described as the "bottom-up" approach. Several other "kits" (Table 6-1) have also become available with minor modifications, including a "top-down" approach whereby the trocars are passed retropubically from the anterior abdominal wall to the vaginal incision, and the tape is attached to the vaginal end of the trocar and then pulled back up through the retropubic space to exit in the suprapubic area.

Indications, Patient Selection, and Types of Slings

The indications for retropubic MUS placement include symptomatic SUI or occult stress incontinence. The initial studies assessing functionality of the retropubic MUS mostly included "ideal" women—ones who were not obese (body mass index >35), who had stress predominant incontinence with a mobile urethra, and who were without prolapse. Preference was for women who had not had prior incontinence procedures (to reduce the risk of bladder perforation during trocar passage). In time, studies also documented excellent outcomes in women who were overweight, had mixed urinary incontinence, had intrinsic sphincter deficiency (ISD) with a lack of urethral hypermobility, and in whom the procedure was performed in conjunction with a vaginal prolapse repair. Retropubic anatomy, prior surgery, and body habitus remain important variables to consider in surgical planning.

Absolute contraindications to the procedure include any important structure potentially in the path of the trocars or sling such as a pelvic kidney or vascular graft, pregnancy, and active oral anticoagulation. Relative contraindications include a history of any condition, such as a ruptured appendix with peritonitis or stage 4 endometriosis, that could put the patient at a high risk of having significant pelvic adhesions, with the risk of small bowel being firmly adhered to the back of the pubic bone. In such circumstances, a transobturator sling would be a preferred procedure because the retropubic space would be completely avoided.

Other patients in whom a synthetic sling is probably inappropriate include patients who are undergoing concurrent or have undergone prior urethral reconstruction. Examples include urethral diverticulectomy, urethrovaginal fistula repair, or urethral injury secondary to prior sling placement or pelvic fracture. Although there are no reports of MUS being used in this setting, experience with synthetic material in the setting of urethral reconstruction has demonstrated a high rate of erosion (Morgan et al., 1985). In contrast, excellent outcomes have been reported with the use of a biologic pubovaginal sling in the setting of reconstruction, with an 88% cure rate after diverticulectomy in 16 patients and an 86% cure rate after genitourinary fistula repair in 7 patients, with no reported erosions (Carey et al., 2002). Also, a synthetic MUS is not recommended in patients with neurogenic incontinence, such as spina bifida, because they are already dependent on clean intermittent self-catheterization, and a tension-free MUS may not provide the necessary compression to achieve continence in between catheterizations. Biologic pubovaginal slings have been used successfully in patients with neurogenic causes of SUI, providing occlusion at the bladder neck, with continence rates in one study of 95% (Austin et al., 2001).

As previously mentioned, the initial TVT system was classified as a bottom-top technique. An alternative system called SPARC (American Medical Systems, Minnetonka, MN) was developed a few years later with the passage of the trocar from the suprapubic region down into the vagina (top-down technique). A meta-analysis by Ogah et al. (2009) compared five randomized controlled trials of TVT versus SPARC and showed that the TVT had higher subjective and objective cure rates of 85% and 92% compared with 77% and 87% of SPARC. The same study showed significantly lower complication rates in the patients receiving TVT (less bladder perforation, mesh erosions, and voiding dysfunction). However, these findings have not been duplicated in other single arm series, which have demonstrated comparable efficacy and low complication rates with the top-down technique (SPARC). Table 6-1 lists the commercially available synthetic retropubic MUS.

> ### Case 1: Primary Stress Incontinence
>
> A 38-year-old woman with bothersome SUI is strongly desirous of surgical intervention. She is gravida 2, para 2, and is still having normal periods but is no longer interested in childbearing.
>
> She has occasional urgency but voids five times per day and experiences urinary loss with activities such as lifting, laughing, and coughing. She uses two moderate thickness pads per day. She has no significant medical conditions and has had no prior pelvic surgery.
>
> On physical examination, she has no abdominal findings. Vaginal examination reveals urethral hypermobility (35 degrees with abdominal straining) and demonstrable loss of urine with coughing while supine with a subjectively empty bladder. No prolapse is noted. Neurologic examination is normal. Although not mandatory, urodynamics studies were performed, and findings were a post-void residual of 30 mL, a stable detrusor on filling cystometry to a maximum of 550 mL, and easily demonstrable urodynamic SUI at 150 mL in the sitting position with Valsalva leak point pressure of 55 cm H_2O.
>
> After a detailed discussion of all management options, the patient decided to proceed with a retropubic synthetic MUS.

Surgical Technique

Bottom-to-Top

1. *Anesthesia.* We prefer to use general anesthesia; however, some surgeons prefer intravenous sedation with local anesthesia to allow the performance of the cough stress test to facilitate appropriate tensioning of the sling. Because approximately 50% of cases are done in conjunction with a prolapse repair, all surgeons need to be well versed at tensioning techniques under general anesthesia (see Step 6).

2. *Vaginal dissection.* The anterior vaginal wall is hydrodistended with a combination of lidocaine and epinephrine, with the goal of completely blanching the anterior vaginal wall at the level of the mid- to distal urethra. A scalpel blade is used to make an incision from just below the external urethral meatus to the level of the midurethra. The vaginal wall is sharply dissected with Metzenbaum scissors off the posterior urethra, creating small tunnels to the inferior pubic ramus. Sharp dissection is required for this dissection because the distal anterior vaginal wall and posterior urethra are fused at this level (Figure 6-2). Some physicians prefer to hydrodissect the trocar trajectory bilaterally before passing the trocars.

3. *Trocar passage.* A catheter guide is placed in the indwelling Foley catheter so that the urethra and bladder neck can be displaced away from where the trocar is inserted. The trocar tip is inserted into the previously dissected tunnel on each side lateral to the urethra and advanced to the undersurface of the pubic bone. The tip of the trocar should be sandwiched between the index finger of the surgeon's nondominant hand placed in the anterior vaginal fornix and the undersurface of the interior pubic ramus. The tip of the needle is carefully advanced through the endopelvic fascia into the retropubic space (Figure 6-3). When the resistance of the endopelvic fascia is overcome and the tip of the needle is in the retropubic space, the handle of the trocar is dropped, and the needle is advanced through the retropubic space as it hugs the back of the pubic bone (Figure 6-4). The next resistance felt is the rectus muscle and anterior abdominal fascia. The needle is advanced through these structures to exit through the previously made

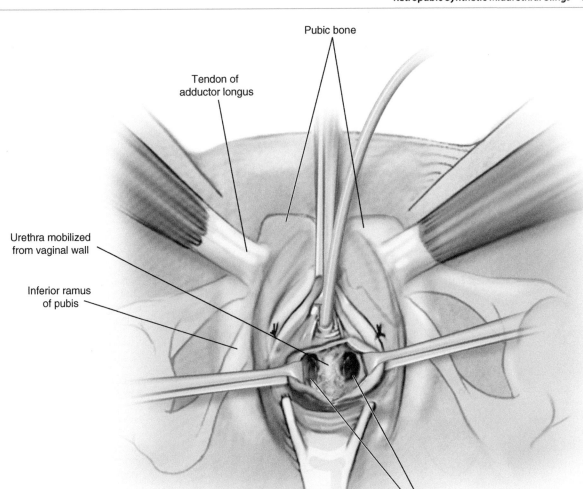

Pubic bone

Tendon of
adductor longus

Urethra mobilized
from vaginal wall

Inferior ramus
of pubis

Tunnels created toward
ipsilateral shoulder of each side

Figure 6-2 Vaginal incision for retropubic midurethral sling. Tunnels are created bilaterally to allow trocars to come into direct contact with the inferior pubic ramus.

suprapubic stab wound (see Figure 6-4). Figures 6-5 and 6-6 illustrate the appropriate passage of the needle through the retropubic space when viewed from above.

4. *Cystoscopy.* Cystoscopy is performed with a 30- or 70-degree scope to evaluate the bladder for inadvertent trocar injury with the trocar in place. If such an injury were to occur, it would generally be visualized in the anterolateral aspect of the bladder (usually the area between 1 o'clock and 3 o'clock on the left side and 9 o'clock and 11 o'clock on the right side). If the trocar is seen or there is any creasing of the bladder mucosa that does not disappear with bladder distention, the trocar should be withdrawn and repassed. Most commonly when the bladder is perforated (which occurs in approximately 3% to 5% of cases), it is because the surgeon has allowed the trocar to migrate away from the back of the pubic bone in a cephalad direction (see Figure 6-5, *A*). During repassing of the trocar, great care should be taken to hug the back of the pubic bone. In such cases, the patient may still proceed with the voiding trial postoperatively without the need for discharge with an indwelling catheter because the bladder perforation is very small and is

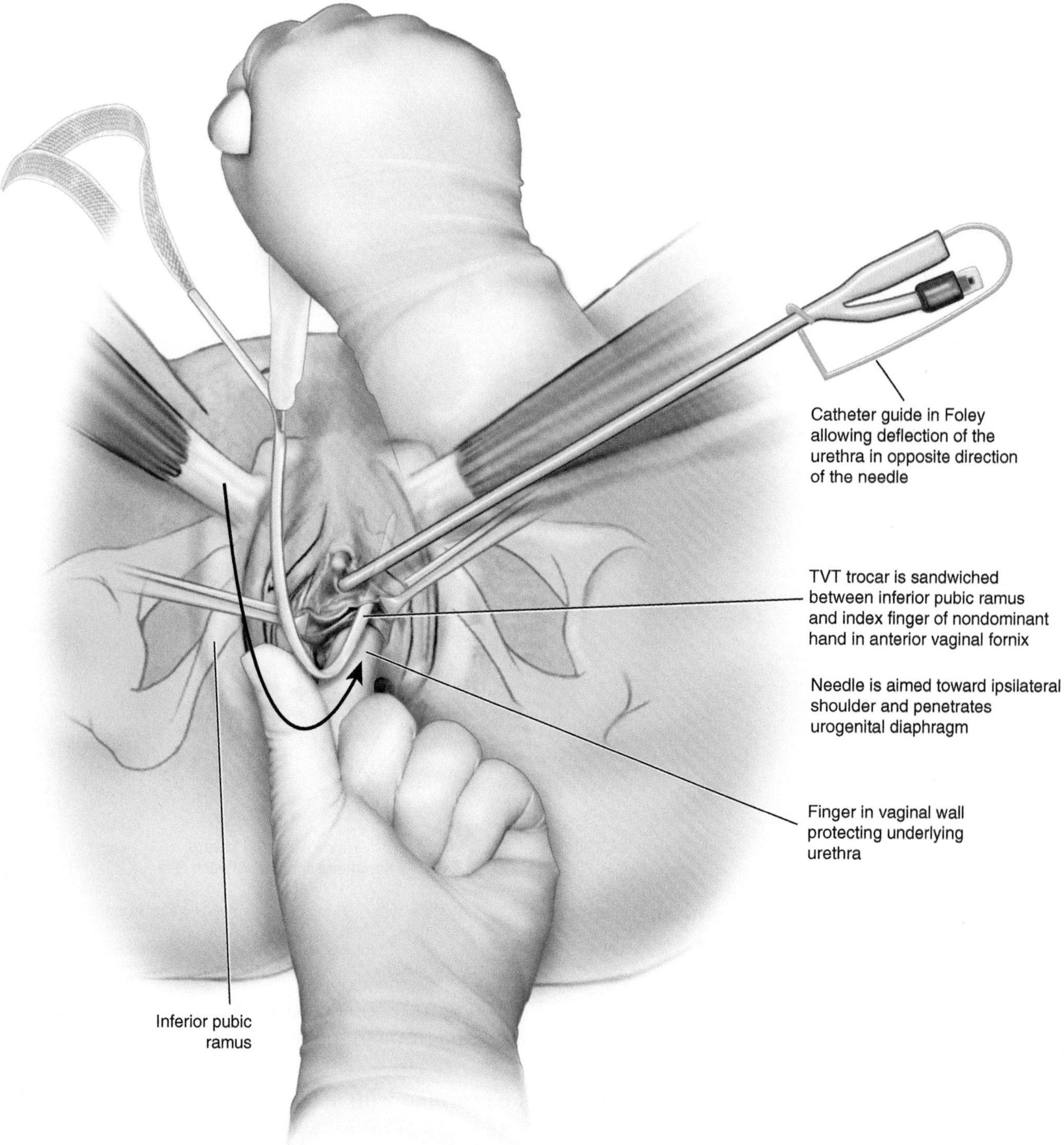

Catheter guide in Foley allowing deflection of the urethra in opposite direction of the needle

TVT trocar is sandwiched between inferior pubic ramus and index finger of nondominant hand in anterior vaginal fornix

Needle is aimed toward ipsilateral shoulder and penetrates urogenital diaphragm

Finger in vaginal wall protecting underlying urethra

Inferior pubic ramus

Figure 6-3 Technique for initial passage of trocars through the vaginal incision into the retropubic space.

usually in a high, nondependent portion of the bladder. If excessive hematuria is present or the perforation is in the base or trigone of the bladder, continuous postoperative bladder drainage should be undertaken.

5. As the ends of the mesh device are attached to the trocars on each side, the mesh with its plastic sheath is pulled up through the suprapubic stab wound along the trocar trajectory.

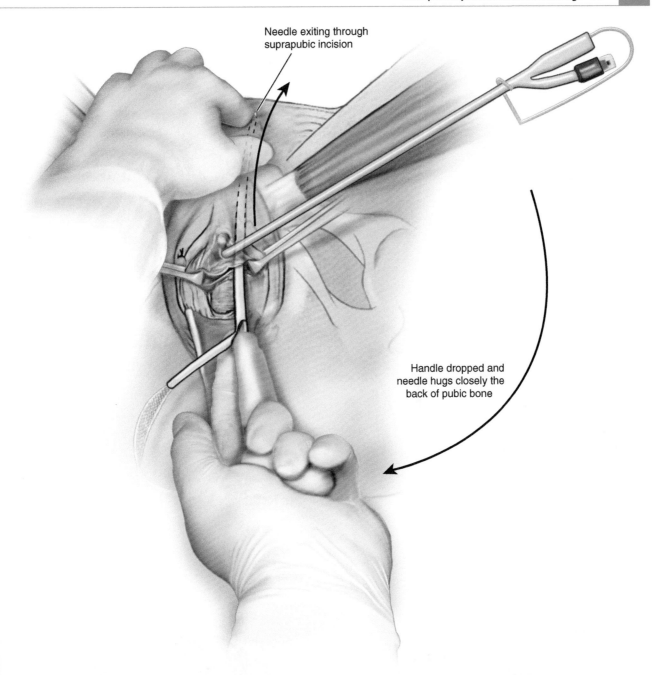

Needle exiting through
suprapubic incision

Handle dropped and
needle hugs closely the
back of pubic bone

Figure 6-4 Technique of passage of trocars through the retropubic space.

6. *Tensioning.* Sling tensioning is very subjective. In general, however, the sling is left very loosely (tension-free) under the urethra. Using a No. 8 Hagar dilator or a right-angled clamp inserted between the posterior urethra and the suburethral portion of the sling will help facilitate appropriate tensioning (Figure 6-7). Some surgeons prefer to perform the procedure under local anesthesia and use a cough stress test. In such situations the sling is tensioned to the point at which minimal leakage occurs during coughing. Regardless of tensioning technique, the ultimate endpoint is to create a laxity in the mesh manifested by a ricochet of the mesh back toward the urethra if pulled on vaginally using a right-angled clamp while also avoiding direct mesh contact with the underside of the urethra. After, the plastic sheaths covering the mesh are removed, and tension of the mesh is rechecked. The

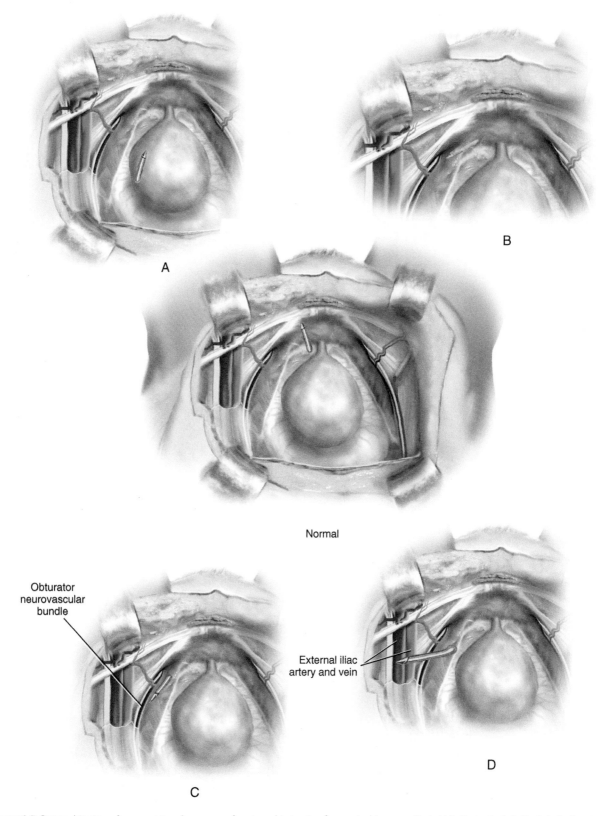

Figure 6-5 Retropubic view of appropriate safe passage of a retropubic tension-free vaginal tape needle *(middle illustration)*. **A,** Cephalad migration of the needle away from the back of the pubic bone is the most common cause of bladder perforation. **B,** External rotation of the handle initially results in penetration of the obturator internus muscle by the needle tip, with the potential to injure aberrant vessels along the lateral pelvic sidewall. **C,** Continued external rotation of the handle with cephalad migration of the needle may result in injury to the obturator neurovascular bundle **(D)** or external iliac vessels.

(From Baggish MS, Karram MM, eds. Atlas of Pelvic Anatomy and Gynecology Surgery, *ed 3. St. Louis: Saunders; 2011.)*

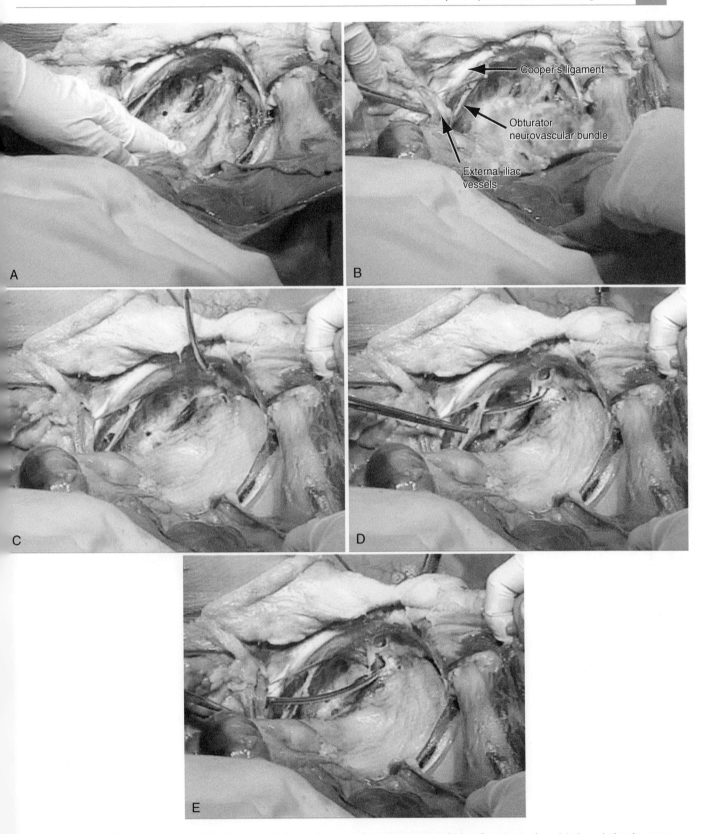

Figure 6-6 A, View of retropubic space of a fresh cadaver. **B,** Cooper ligament, obturator neurovascular bundle as it exits the pelvis through the obturator foramen, and external iliac vessels as they exit the pelvis under the inguinal ligament are marked. **C,** A tension-free vaginal tape (TVT) needle has been passed in an appropriate fashion on the left side of this cadaver. **D,** The TVT needle is intentionally continued in a cephalad-lateral direction, and one can see how it can easily come into contact with the obturator neurovascular bundle in the retropubic space. **E,** The TVT needle is intentionally continued in this direction, and one can see how it could potentially come in contact with the external iliac vessels.

(From Baggish MS, Karram MM, eds. Atlas of Pelvic Anatomy and Gynecology Surgery, *ed 3. St. Louis: Saunders; 2011.)*

Figure 6-7 Technique for tensioning sling.

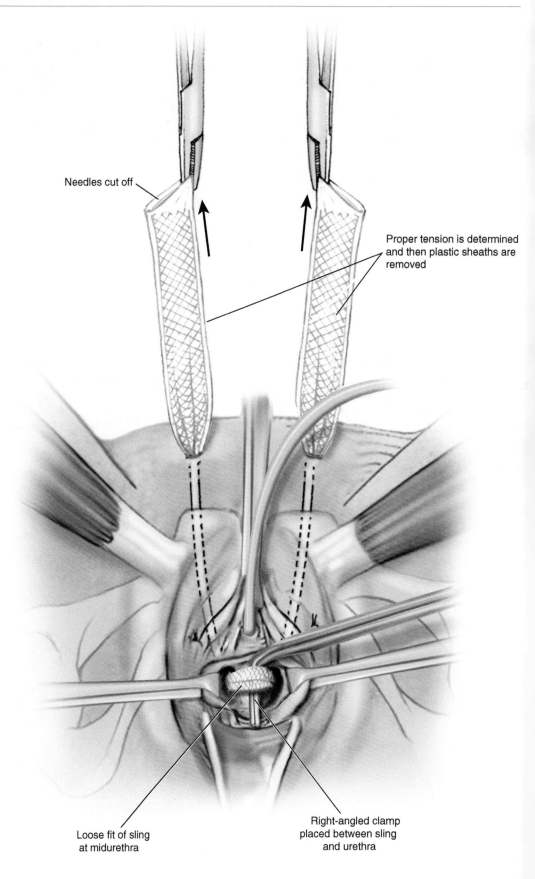

Needles cut off

Proper tension is determined and then plastic sheaths are removed

Loose fit of sling at midurethra

Right-angled clamp placed between sling and urethra

mesh is resected flush with the skin suprapubically, making sure to mobilize the skin away from the mesh ends before skin closure (see Figure 6-7).

7. The vaginal wound is copiously irrigated and closed with a running 3-0 polyglycolic acid suture. The suprapubic stab wounds are closed with absorbable suture or liquid tissue adhesive. Vaginal packing may be inserted temporarily at the completion of the case if the patient is bleeding or concurrent prolapse procedures are being performed.

8. The catheter may be removed along with the vaginal packing in the recovery room, and the patient is discharged after confirming voiding efficiency (**Videos 6-1** and **6-2**).

Top-to-Bottom

1. *Vaginal dissection.* The vaginal incision should be larger than described for the bottom-to-top technique because the dissection should allow placement of the index finger of the surgeon's nondominant hand into the incision so as to pick up the tip of the needle as it passes into the vaginal incision (Figure 6-8).

2. *Top-to-bottom trocar passage.* Before passage of the trocars, complete drainage of the bladder is ensured. At the previously marked puncture sites in the suprapubic region, a stab incision is made on each side. The incisions should be well within the pubic tubercles bilaterally. A trocar is inserted into the first of the suprapubic incisions while aligning with the sagittal axis of the body and then carefully puncturing through the anterior rectus sheath. By angling caudally and "walking off" the superior posterior edge of the pubic bone, the trocar is advanced into the retropubic space maintaining close contact with the posterior surface of the pubic bone. Concurrently, the surgeon's finger is inserted into the previously dissected periurethral space on the ipsilateral side to provide control of the distal tip of the trocar. In a controlled manner, the trocar is progressively advanced until the tip is visible in the vaginal incision. Cystoscopy as previously described is performed to confirm that the needle did not penetrate the bladder. The same maneuver is performed on the contralateral side (Figures 6-9 and 6-10).

3. *Loading of the mesh.* The mesh is attached to the trocars, and the trocars are withdrawn through the suprapubic stab wounds. Tensioning of the sling is as previously described for the bottom-to-top technique (**Video 6-3** ; see Figure 6-7).

Outcomes of Retropubic Synthetic Midurethral Slings

The Cochrane Library published a meta-analysis (based on 62 studies) showing short-term cure rates for retropubic MUS to be between 73% and 82% (Bezerra and Bruschini 2005). The largest randomized controlled study comparing retropubic and transobturator slings (Trial of Mid-Urethral Slings [TOMUS]) showed retropubic sling subjective and objective cure rates to be 62% and 78%, respectively (Richter et al., 2010). Two prospective cohort studies reporting 7-year and 11-year follow-up after TVT slings reported subjective cure rates of 85% and 77%, respectively (Nilsson et al., 2008).

A Cochrane review in 2009 (Ogah, Cody, and Rogerson, 2009) compared retropubic MUS based on insertion techniques and showed a statistically significant difference with benefit for the bottom-to-top approach. This review was based on five trials and showed evidence of lower erosion rates, bladder

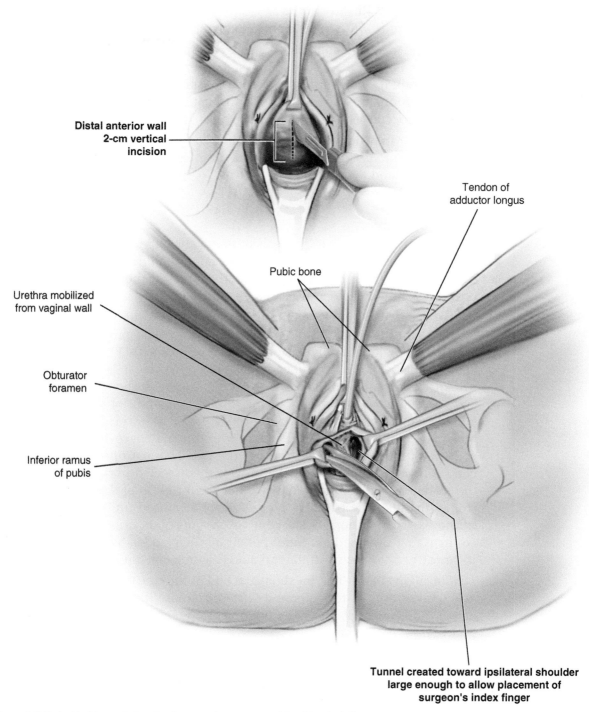

Distal anterior wall 2-cm vertical incision

Tendon of adductor longus

Pubic bone

Urethra mobilized from vaginal wall

Obturator foramen

Inferior ramus of pubis

Tunnel created toward ipsilateral shoulder large enough to allow placement of surgeon's index finger

Figure 6-8 Vaginal incision and dissection for top-to-bottom retropubic midurethral sling.

perforations, and postoperative voiding dysfunction with the bottom-to-top technique. However, the difference in perioperative complications overall was not statistically significant. When comparing retropubic MUS with laparoscopic colposuspension, there was no difference in incontinence cure rates among the two groups; however, blood loss was significantly less in the sling group. Studies comparing retropubic MUS with open colposuspension procedures (the 2005 Cochrane review [Bezerra and Bruschini 2005] and the Ward trial with 5-year follow-up [Ward et al., 2008]) showed similar cure rates with both techniques.

Although there is no standardized definition, ISD has been defined in the literature based on the urodynamics findings of Valsalva leak point pressure of

Figure 6-9 Technique for passage of top-to-bottom trocar through vaginal incision.

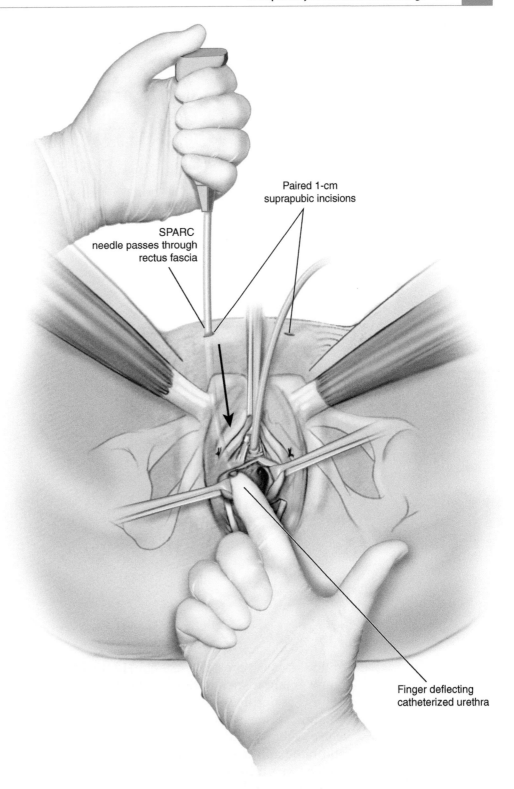

Paired 1-cm suprapubic incisions

SPARC needle passes through rectus fascia

Finger deflecting catheterized urethra

less than 60 cm H_2O or maximum urethral closure pressure of less than 20 cm H_2O. Women with ISD have been reported to have more severe incontinence with higher risk of treatment failure. Before the development of synthetic sling kits, biologic bladder neck slings had been recommended in such cases with reported cure rates of 80% to 85%. Numerous studies to date have reported good success with retropubic TVT in women with ISD. Rezapour et al. (2001) first reported their results using TVT in 49 women with ISD (defined maximum

Figure 6-10 Side view illustrating how top-to-bottom trocar should hug back of pubic bone.

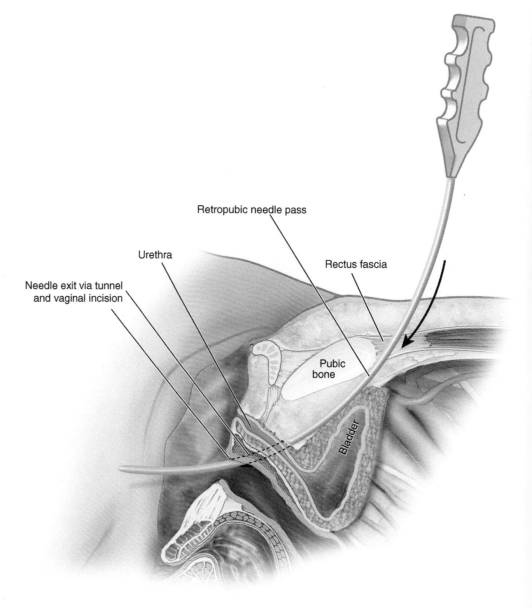

Retropubic needle pass

Urethra

Needle exit via tunnel and vaginal incision

Rectus fascia

Pubic bone

Bladder

Side view

urethral closure pressure <20 cm H_2O) with a cure rate of 74% and significant improvement in an additional 12% of cases. Of the seven failures, five had fixed urethras as defined by a Q-tip test of <30%. Although the numbers were small, the authors suggested that lack of urethral mobility may be a risk factor for failure. Subsequently, numerous studies have compared retropubic with transobturator approaches in patients with ISD using the previously mentioned urodynamics criteria. Jeon et al. (2008) retrospectively compared TVT, transobturator tape, and pubovaginal sling in women with ISD followed for 2 years. Patients with TVT had a cure rate of 86.9%, which was similar to the cure rate of 87.3% seen with the pubovaginal sling; in contrast, the transobturator tape group had a cure rate of only 34.9% ($P < .0001$). At 31 months, Gungorduk et al. (2009) found cure rates of 78.3% using TVT versus 52.5% using transobturator slings and concluded that transobturator slings were five times more likely to fail than TVT in women with ISD. In the only prospective, randomized study addressing this issue, Schierlitz et al. (2008) randomly assigned 164 women with ISD to TVT or TOT, with the primary outcome of urodynamic SUI at 6 months being that 21% of the TVT group had SUI versus 45% of the TOT group ($P = .004$). Also, 13% of women in the TOT group requested repeat slings compared with none in the TVT group.

This literature suggests that retropubic slings work well for patients with ISD, whereas transobturator slings may not work as well. In contrast, a retrospective study by Rapp et al. (2009) found no difference between retropubic and transobturator slings in women with ISD with success rates of 76% and 77%, respectively. Constantini et al. (2008) also reported no difference between TVT and TOT in women with ISD, using a subset analysis of their randomized controlled trial; however, all of their patients had urethral hypermobility ranging from 43 degrees to 90 degrees on the Q-tip test. They found no difference in outcomes between 45 patients with TVT and 50 patients with TOT at 35 months (68% vs. 76%). Although this was a post-hoc analysis that was underpowered to detect a difference, it does suggest that patients with ISD who have concurrent hypermobility may show similar outcomes with both TVT and TOT slings.

A study by Haliloglu et al. (2010) examined the impact of ISD and urethral hypermobility in 65 patients with transobturator tape by dividing them into three groups: ISD with hypermobility (n = 18), ISD with fixed urethra (n = 16), and hypermobility without ISD (n = 31). At 24 months, the two groups with hypermobility had similar cure rates, with and without ISD (87.5% and 96.4%). However, patients with no hypermobility had a significantly lower cure rate (66.7%). Hypermobility was also a predictive factor in patients undergoing TVT in a series reported by Fritel et al. (2002) with success rates of 92% for Q-tip test greater than 30 degrees versus 70% for Q-tip test less than 30 degrees. ISD, which was defined in this study as a maximum urethral closure pressure less than 20 cm H_2O, had no impact on success rate. The literature seems to indicate retropubic and transobturator MUS procedures are effective in treating patients with ISD and hypermobility; however, the less mobile urethra is a risk factor for transobturator sling failure, and a retropubic approach may be favored in these cases.

Complications

Complications of retropubic MUS procedures include bladder perforation, pelvic visceral injuries, vascular injuries and hemorrhage, mesh erosion and extrusion, de novo development of urgency and urge incontinence, bladder outlet obstruction, and urinary tract infection.

Bladder perforation is simply managed by trocar removal and reinsertion. However, if a large injury has been encountered in a dependent portion of the bladder (trigone or bladder base), prolonged drainage or rarely aborting the procedure is recommended. Mesh immediately adjacent to a bladder injury can result in erosion into the urinary tract. Studies have shown that experience plays a major role in trocar perforation rates, with rates as low as 1% in experienced hands and as high as 35% in the hands of novice surgeons. If urethral injury is noted, the procedure is preferably abandoned until complete healing has occurred to reduce the likelihood of erosions of mesh into the urethra. See Chapter 14 for a more detailed discussion of avoiding and managing such complications. Bleeding, depending on the amount, may indicate trocar injury to pelvic vessels including accessory obturator vessels, paravesical vessels, circumflex or inferior epigastric vessels, and in rare situations external iliac or femoral vessels. Sometimes this bleeding may be concealed and result in a large hematoma, with the only postoperative symptoms being a subjective feeling of discomfort, pressure, or frequency of urination. Objective indicators include a drop in blood pressure, tachycardia, oliguria, a palpable suprapubic mass, and loss of consciousness in extreme cases. One study showed a correlation between hematoma size and symptoms, with the patient in severe discomfort if the collection was larger than 300 mL compared with minimal to absent symptoms at volumes less than 100 mL. Persistent bleeding refractory to passive actions such as compression and active modalities such as hemagglutinants may require angiographic management and vascular surgical consultation. Management of postoperative voiding dysfunction and retention are discussed in Chapter 9.

Retropubic MUS may also result in pain, which may be experienced in the suprapubic or vaginal areas. Although often transient, persistent pain after mesh implantation can rarely result in significant morbidity and patient quality of life disturbance. Sling tensioning may play a role in the de novo development of pain. First-line therapy is based on optimization of analgesia and use of antiinflammatory medications. Local anesthetic injections and more advanced pain management may be necessary. A final intervention is surgical excision of the sling, which results in resolution or improvement of pain in 50% to 68% of the patients. If the suburethral portion of the sling is excised, recurrent SUI will usually develop in at least 30% of cases. Dyspareunia can occur and is often related to superficial mesh location (inclusive of mesh exposure). Although topical vaginal estrogen application and observation have been advocated for this problem, most patients require mesh removal for symptom resolution (see Chapter 14).

Mesh erosion and extrusion is a known complication of all synthetic mesh systems. In a series of 241 women, Abouassaly et al. (2004) reported a 1% vaginal erosion rate after TVT. Initial treatment after diagnosis is typically conservative with use of vaginal estrogen cream and avoidance of vaginal insertions or trauma including pelvic rest and avoiding intercourse. If conservative treatment is unsuccessful, surgical options include mobilization and reapproximation of vaginal epithelium over the exposed mesh, excision of the exposed mesh, or complete removal of the suburethral portion of the mesh in more severe cases. Removal of the mesh should be done only after adequate patient counseling relative to the likelihood of recurrence of SUI.

Obesity and Retropubic Slings

Both safety and effectiveness are important when assessing any surgical procedures. Multiple studies have reported no significant difference in outcomes in obese patients undergoing retropubic MUS on long-term follow-up. However, a meta-analysis in 2008 did show a statistically significant difference in SUI cure rates (81% in obese patients versus 85% in nonobese patients). De novo urge incontinence was not noted to vary between the two groups, but the rate of persistent urge incontinence was significantly higher in obese patients. When comparing safety, the same meta-analysis showed that obese patients had a statistically significant lower bladder perforation rate (Greer, Richter, Bartolucci, and Burgio, 2008).

Pregnancy After Retropubic Slings

In the authors' opinion, whenever possible, SUI surgery should be delayed until the completion of childbirth. If a synthetic sling is placed in a woman who eventually becomes pregnant, there are insufficient data at the present time to support abdominal versus vaginal delivery. Because of the stretch and pressure generated during labor and pregnancy, there is a concern that the support offered by synthetic slings may be impacted negatively with subsequent loss of adequate urinary control postpartum. A case series by Groenen et al. (2008) reported a more favorable outcome related to maintenance of continence after cesarean sections versus vaginal delivery.

Conclusion

Both subjective and objective long-term cure rates for retropubic MUS appear to be high with minimal complications reported regardless of body habitus, the presence of ISD, and recurrent SUI. Ultimately, the appropriate continence procedure to be performed should be selected by both the patient and the physician after discussion of all risks, cures rates, and patient expectations.

Suggested Readings

Abouassaly R, Steinberg JR, Lemieux M, et al. Complications of tension-free vaginal tape surgery: multi-institutional review. *BJU Int.* 2004;94:110-113.

Austin PF, Westney OL, Leng WW, et al. Advantages of rectus fascial slings for urinary incontinence in children with neuropathic bladders. *J Urol.* 2001;165:2369-2371.

Bezerra CA, Bruschini H. Suburethral sling operations for urinary incontinence in women. *Cochrane Database Syst Rev.* 2001;(3):CD001754. [Update in *Cochrane Database Syst Rev.* 2005;(3):CD001754.]

Blaivas JG, Sandhu J. Urethral reconstruction after erosion of slings in women. *Curr Opin Urol.* 2004;14:335-338.

Bodelsson G, Henriksson L, Osser S, Stjernquist M. Short term complications of the tension free vaginal tape operation for stress urinary incontinence in women. *Br J Obstet Gynaecol.* 2002;109:566-569.

Carey MP, Goh JT, Fynes MM, et al. Stress urinary incontinence after delayed primary closure of genitourinary fistula: a technique for surgical management. *Am J Obstet Gynecol.* 2002;186:948-953.

Constantini E, Lazzeri M, Giannantoni A, et al. Preoperative Valsalva leak point pressure may not predict outcome of mid-urethral slings: analysis from a randomized controlled trial of retropubic versus transobturator mid-urethral slings. *Int Braz J Urol.* 2008;34:73-81.

Duckett JR, Patil A, Papanikolaou NS. Predicting early voiding dysfunction after tension-free vaginal tape. *J Obstet Gynaecol.* 2008;28:89-92.

Flock F, Reich A, Muche R, Kreienberg R, Reister F. Hemorrhagic complications associated with tension-free vaginal tape procedure. *Obstet Gynecol.* 2004;104(5 Pt 1):989-994.

Fong ED, Nitti VW. Review article: Mid-urethral synthetic slings for female stress urinary incontinence. *BJU Int.* 2010;106:596-608.

Fritel X, Zabak K, Pigne A, et al. Predictive value of urethral mobility before suburethral tape procedure for urinary stress incontinence in women. *J Urol.* 2002;168:2472-2475.

Greer WJ, Richter HE, Bartolucci AA, Burgio KL. Obesity and pelvic floor disorders: a systematic review. *Obstet Gynecol.* 2008;112:341-349.

Groenen R, Vos MC, Willekes C, Vervest HA. Pregnancy and delivery after mid-urethral sling procedures for stress urinary incontinence: case reports and a review of literature. *Int Urogynecol J Pelvic Floor Dysfunct.* 2008;19:441-448.

Gungorduk K, Celebi I, Ark C, et al. Which type of mid-urethral sling procedure should be chosen for treatment of stress urinary incontinence with intrinsic sphincter deficiency? Tension-free vaginal tape or transobturator tape. *Acta Obstet Gynecol Scand.* 2009;88:920-926.

Haliloglu B, Karateke A, Coksuer H, Peker H, Cam C. The role of urethral hypermobility and intrinsic sphincteric deficiency on the outcome of transobturator tape procedure: a prospective study with 2-year follow-up. *Int Urogynecol J.* 2010;21:173-178.

Jang HC, Jeon JH, Kim DY. Changes in sexual function after the midurethral sling procedure for stress urinary incontinence: long-term follow-up. *Int Neurourol J.* 2010;14:170-176.

Jeffry L, Deval B, Birsan A, Soriano D, Daraï E. Objective and subjective cure rates after tension-free vaginal tape for treatment of urinary incontinence. *Urology.* 2001;58:702-706.

Jeon M-J, Jung H-J, Chung S-M, Kim S-K, Bai S-W. Comparison of the treatment outcome of pubovaginal sling, tension-free vaginal tape, and transobturator tape for stress urinary incontinence with intrinsic sphincter deficiency. *Am J Obstet Gynecol.* 2008;199:76.e1-76.e4.

Koops SE, Bisseling TM, van Brummen HJ, Heintz AP, Vervest HA. What determines a successful tension-free vaginal tape? A prospective multicenter cohort study: results from The Netherlands TVT database. *Am J Obstet Gynecol.* 2006;194:65-74.

Liapis A, Bakas P, Creatsas G. Tension-free vaginal tape in the management of recurrent urodynamic stress incontinence after previous failed midurethral tape. *Eur Urol.* 2009;55:1450-1455.

Lim JL, de Cuyper EM, Cornish A, Frazer M. Short-term clinical and quality-of-life outcomes in women treated by the TVT-Secur procedure. *Aust N Z J Obstet Gynaecol.* 2010;50:168-172.

Lovatsis D, Easton W, Wilkie D. Guidelines for the evaluation and treatment of recurrent urinary incontinence following pelvic floor surgery. Society of Obstetricians and Gynaecologists of Canada Urogynaecology Committee. *J Obstet Gynaecol Can.* 2010;32:893-904.

Morgan JE, Farrow GA, Stewart FE. The Marlex sling operation for the treatment of recurrent stress urinary incontinence: a 16-year review. *Am J Obstet Gynecol.* 1985;151:224-226.

Morton HC, Hilton P. Urethral injury associated with minimally invasive mid-urethral sling procedures for the treatment of stress urinary incontinence: a case series and systematic literature search. *Br J Obstet Gynaecol.* 2009;116:1120-1126.

Nilsson CG, Palva K, Rezapour M, Falconer C. Eleven years prospective follow-up of the tension-free vaginal tape procedure for treatment of stress urinary incontinence. *Int Urogynecol J Pelvic Floor Dysfunct.* 2008;19:1043-1047.

Ogah J, Cody DJ, Rogerson L. Minimally invasive synthetic suburethral sling operations for stress urinary incontinence in women: a short version Cochrane review. *Neurourol Urodyn.* 2011;30: 284-291.

Ogah J, Cody JD, Rogerson L. Minimally invasive synthetic suburethral sling operations for stress urinary incontinence in women. *Cochrane Database Syst Rev.* 2009;(4):CD006375.

Panel L, Triopon G, Courtieu C, Marès P, de Tayrac R. How to advise a woman who wants to get pregnant after a sub-urethral tape placement? *Int Urogynecol J Pelvic Floor Dysfunct.* 2008;19:347-350.

Rafii A, Daraï E, Haab F, Samain E, Levardon M, Deval B. Body mass index and outcome of tension-free vaginal tape. *Eur Urol.* 2003;43:288-292.

Rapp DE, Govier FE, Kobashi KC. Outcomes following mid-urethral sling placement in patients with intrinsic sphincteric deficiency: comparison of SPARC and MONARC slings. *Int Braz J Urol.* 2009;35:68-75.

Rehman H, Bezerra CC, Bruschini H, Cody JD. Traditional suburethral sling operations for urinary incontinence in women. *Cochrane Database Syst Rev.* 2011;(1):CD001754.

Rezapour M, Falconer C, Ulmsten U. Tension-free vaginal tape (TVT) in stress incontinent women with intrinsic sphincter deficiency (ISD)—a long term follow-up. *Int Urogynecol J Pelvic Floor Dysfunct.* 2001;12(Suppl 2):S12-S14.

Richter HE, Albo ME, Zyczynski HM, et al; Urinary Incontinence Treatment Network. Retropubic versus transobturator midurethral slings for stress incontinence. *N Engl J Med.* 2010;362: 2066-2076.

Rigaud J, Pothin P, Labat JJ, et al. Functional results after tape removal for chronic pelvic pain following tension-free vaginal tape or transobturator tape. *J Urol.* 2010;184:610-615.

Schierlitz L, Dwyer PL, Rosamilia A, et al. Effectiveness of tension-free vaginal tape compared with transobturator tape in women with stress urinary incontinence and intrinsic sphincter deficiency: a randomized controlled trial. *Obstet Gynecol.* 2008;112:1253-1261.

Ulmsten U, Petros P. Intravaginal slingplasty (IVS): an ambulatory surgical procedure for treatment of female urinary incontinence. *Scand J Urol Nephrol.* 1995;29:75-82.

Wang AC. The techniques of trocar insertion and intraoperative urethrocystoscopy in tension-free vaginal taping: an experience of 600 cases. *Acta Obstet Gynecol Scand.* 2004;83:293.

Ward KL, Hilton P; UK and Ireland TVT Trial Group. Tension-free vaginal tape versus colposuspension for primary urodynamic stress incontinence: 5-year follow up. *Br J Obstet Gynaecol.* 2008; 115:226-233.

Transobturator Synthetic Midurethral Slings

7

Dani Zoorob, M.D.
Mickey Karram, M.D.

 Videos

7-1 Transobturator Sling: Inside-Out Technique (Example 1)
7-2 Transobturator Sling: Inside-Out Technique (Example 2)

7-3 Transobturator Sling: Outside-In Technique (MONARC)

Introduction

Because retropubic midurethral slings require blind passage of a trocar through the retropubic space, inadvertent bladder perforation occurs in 3% to 5% of cases. Also, vascular and bowel injuries, albeit very rare, were reported that resulted in significant morbidity and mortality (see Chapter 6). In the hope of avoiding these complications, Delorme described the transobturator technique for midurethral sling placement in 2001.

As with retropubic synthetic slings, this is a minimally invasive midurethral sling using a synthetic tape; however, it is placed using a transobturator approach rather than a retropubic one, almost eliminating any potential for bladder or bowel perforation and major vascular injury. Specially designed needles are passed either from the inner groin into the vaginal incision (outside-in technique) or from the vaginal incision into the inner groin (inside-out technique). When the procedure is performed in an appropriate fashion, the needle and subsequently the sling pass through (from outside in) the subcutaneous fat, gracilis tendon, adductor brevis, obturator externus, obturator membrane, and obturator internus. (See Chapter 3 for a detailed discussion of obturator anatomy.) Transobturator tape (TOT) slings use the basic concept of midurethral support with the sling placed underneath the urethra; resistance against the urethra is generated when intra-abdominal pressure increases, which increases outlet resistance and prevents stress urinary incontinence (SUI).

TOT slings have become the most popular surgical treatment for SUI. The technique has been shown to be a low-risk procedure that is comparable to most other surgical options in effectiveness.

TOT slings are associated with a lower risk of urethral obstruction, urinary retention, and subsequent need for sling release compared with retropubic slings. For primary cases, a TOT sling demonstrates similar rates of cure compared with retropubic synthetic slings, with fewer bladder perforations and postoperative irritative voiding symptoms. Also, as mentioned, rare but

Table 7-1 Commercially available transobturator midurethral sling kits

Sling	Manufacturer	Trocar Passage
TVT-O	Gynecare, Somerville, NJ	Inside-out
TVT-Abbrevo	Gynecare	Inside-out
Monarc	American Medical Systems, Minnetonka, MN	Outside-in
Obtryx	Boston Scientific Corp, Natick, MA	Outside-in
Align TO	CR Bard, Murray Hill, NJ	Outside-in
Aris	Coloplast, Minneapolis, MN	Outside-in

catastrophic risks of bowel and major vessel injury are almost eliminated. The trade-off is that patients experience more complications referable to the groin, such as pain and leg weakness or numbness, with the TOT approach. Retropubic slings may be more effective for recurrent incontinence and in women with intrinsic sphincter deficiency (ISD), although the data supporting this statement are difficult to interpret owing to controversy regarding how best to define and diagnose ISD.

This chapter reviews the technique for transobturator sling placement and discusses potential complications and outcomes. Numerous transobturator sling kits are available at the present time (Table 7-1). Indications for TOT sling placement include patients with symptomatic SUI or mixed incontinence in which the stress component is more severe than the urge component. TOT slings are also commonly placed in women undergoing repair of pelvic organ prolapse in the hope of preventing the de novo development of SUI (occult incontinence).

Case 1: Primary Stress Incontinence

A 42-year-old woman with symptoms of SUI that significantly impact her quality of life is desirous of definitive surgical treatment. She is gravida 4, para 3, and has had global endometrial ablation. She reports urinary leakage with jogging, sneezing, and laughter and denies any significant urgency or urge incontinence. Her leakage on average requires three protective pads per day. She reports no significant surgical or medical history.

General physical and neurologic examinations are unremarkable. Pelvic examination reveals good support of her uterus and anterior and posterior vaginal walls. Q-tip test notes urethral mobility to 40 degrees with abdominal straining. She has good pelvic muscle contraction and has undergone a course of pelvic floor physical therapy with no significant improvement in SUI. The sign of stress incontinence is easily demonstrable with coughing in the sitting position. Her post-void residual volume is 20 mL and is negative on dipstick.

After a detailed discussion of all surgical options, the patient decided to proceed with a transobturator sling.

Surgical Technique

As previously mentioned, TOT slings can be placed inside-to-outside or outside-to-inside. The indications, effectiveness, and frequency of complications seem to be similar between the two groups (Novara et al., 2010). One study found a higher frequency of de novo sexual dysfunction secondary to the sling being palpable and tender, creating penile pain in the male partner after the outside-in approach (Scheiner et al., 2012). However, this complication has not been observed in all studies (Sentilhes et al., 2009). At the present time, the decision

Figure 7-1 Photograph illustrates the exit point for an inside-out TOT procedure, specifically the TVT-O procedure. The exit point is 2 cm lateral from the labial fold and 2 cm above the level of the urethra.

(From Baggish MS, Karram MM, eds. Atlas of Pelvic Anatomy and Gynecology Surgery, *ed 3. St. Louis: Saunders; 2011.)*

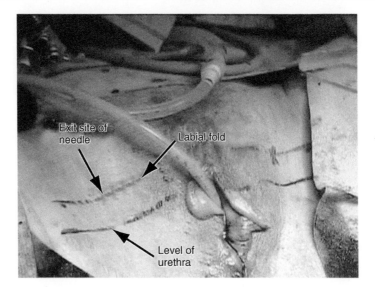

regarding which approach to use is based mostly on how a surgeon was initially trained to perform these procedures.

Inside-Out Technique

1. Preoperative considerations include antibiotic administration for skin and vaginal flora coverage. The antibiotic classes commonly used include intravenous cephalosporins and fluoroquinolones.

2. Sterile urine should be confirmed before the procedure; some physicians postpone the surgery if an active urinary tract infection is documented.

3. *Patient positioning and preparation.* The patient is positioned in the dorsal lithotomy position with legs supported in Allen or candy cane stirrups with all pressure points padded appropriately. The perineum and vagina are sterilely prepared, and surgical draping is placed so as to allow access to the vagina and inner groin.

4. *Anesthesia.* Although the authors prefer to perform these procedures under general anesthesia, they can be performed using intravenous sedation with local infiltration of the vaginal tissue, which allows the use of a cough test to assist in appropriate tensioning of the sling.

5. The exit site of the needle is marked. It should be 2 cm above the level of the urethra and 2 cm lateral to the labial fold (Figures 7-1 and 7-2).

6. *Vaginal incision.* Anterior retraction of the vaginal mucosa with an Allis clamp facilitates visualization. We prefer to hydrodistend the anterior vaginal wall with either a combination of epinephrine and lidocaine or injectable grade saline. A scalpel blade is used to make a distal anterior vaginal wall incision.

7. *Vaginal dissection.* Sharp dissection is used to mobilize the anterior vaginal wall off the underlying urethra. The authors prefer to make the incision slightly longer for TOT and single incision slings than the incision required for retropubic midurethral sling. We prefer to mobilize the distal anterior vaginal wall completely off the posterior urethra allowing placement of the surgeon's finger into the paraurethral space for palpation of the inferior pubic ramus (Figure 7-3). Some physicians prefer to hydrodissect the trocar trajectory bilaterally before placing the sling and its trocar.

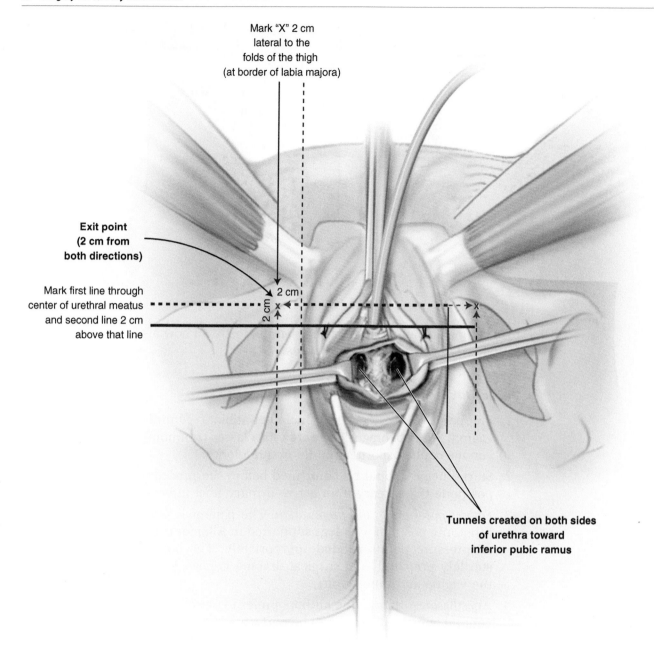

Mark "X" 2 cm
lateral to the
folds of the thigh
(at border of labia majora)

Exit point
(2 cm from
both directions)

Mark first line through
center of urethral meatus
and second line 2 cm
above that line

2 cm

2 cm

Tunnels created on both sides
of urethra toward
inferior pubic ramus

Figure 7-2 Vaginal incision and exit point for the inside-out transobturator sling.

8. *Trocar passage.* The trocar tip is inserted into the previously dissected vaginal incision lateral to the urethra and advanced gently while rotating the trocar handle. This insertion is done while hugging the pubic rami knowing that the obturator canal, which houses both obturator nerve and vessels, is at the opposite anterolateral margin of the foramen. The tip should emerge at the level of the exit site generated previously at the level of the clitoris. The vaginal sulcus is inspected to ensure no perforation or mucosal damage has occurred. Certain TOT sling kits (TVT-O [Gynecare, Somerville, NJ] and TVT-Abbrevo [Gynecare]) have a winged guide introducer that helps facilitate appropriate passage of the needle through the obturator membrane easily guiding the trocar into position. Some surgeons prefer perforating the membrane with Metzerbaum scissors before passing the trocar (Figure 7-4). Once the membrane is penetrated with the tip of

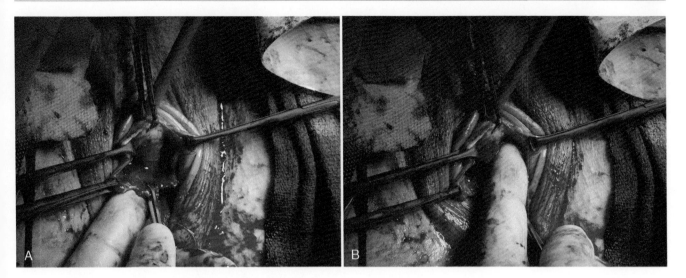

Figure 7-3 A, Anterior vaginal wall incision for a transobturator sling should involve complete mobilization of the distal anterior vaginal wall off the posterior urethra. **B,** The incision should be large enough to allow placement of the surgeon's index finger.

(From Baggish MS, Karram MM, eds. Atlas of Pelvic Anatomy and Gynecology Surgery, ed 3. St. Louis: Saunders; 2011.)

the trocar, the surgeon's hand is lowered or dropped toward the patient to allow the helical trocar to rotate around the ischiopubic ramus and exit in the inner thigh (Figure 7-5).

9. *Cystourethroscopy.* Careful cystoscopy of the urethra and the bladder should be performed to rule out bladder perforation. If the trocar were to perforate the bladder, it would generally be visualized in the anterolateral aspect of the bladder (usually the area between 3 o'clock and 5 o'clock on the left side and 7 o'clock and 9 o'clock on the right side). If the trocar is seen in the bladder, it should be withdrawn and reinserted. Occurrence of bladder or urethral perforation or injury is extremely rare during TOT placement.

10. *Tensioning.* The sling should lay flat against the urethra easily allowing the passage of a right-angled clamp between the sling and the posterior urethra. We prefer to tension TOT slings slightly tighter than retropubic midurethral slings (Figure 7-6).

11. The vaginal wound is copiously irrigated and closed with a running No. 3-0 polyglycolic acid suture. The groin stab wounds are closed with absorbable suture or covered with liquid tissue adhesive. If desired, a vaginal packing may be inserted temporarily at the completion of the case (if the patient is bleeding or concurrent prolapse procedures are being performed).

12. The catheter may be removed (along with the vaginal packing, if present) in the recovery room, and the patient is discharged after documenting voiding efficiency. If unable to void, the patient is taught intermittent self-catheterization or an indwelling Foley catheter is placed (**Video 7-1**).

The TVT-Abbrevo is the most recent version of the inside-out TOT sling. It differs from earlier slings in that the sling is only 12 cm long (vs. traditional 20-cm-long TOT sling). The shorter mesh traverses only the obturator internus, obturator membrane, and obturator externus avoiding all the other inner groin muscles. Nonabsorbable polypropylene (Prolene) sutures are attached to the lateral edges of the mesh to allow for adjustments in mesh tensioning. Also, a

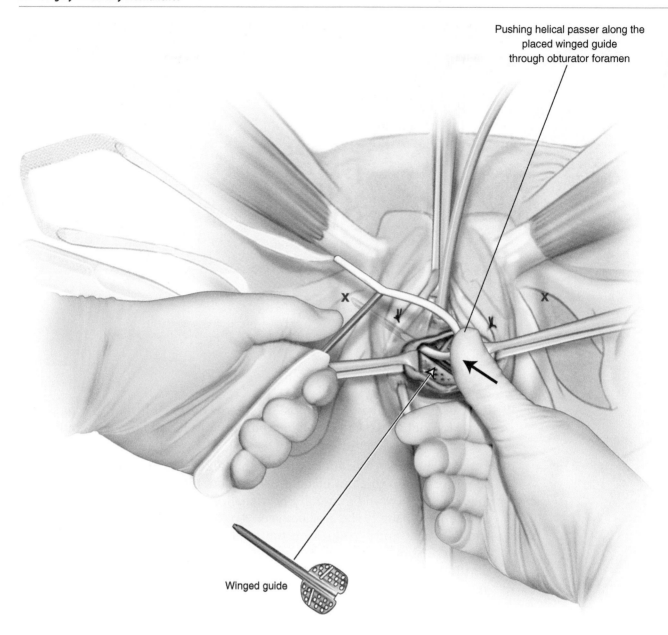

Pushing helical passer along the placed winged guide through obturator foramen

Winged guide

Figure 7-4 Technique for passage of TOT trocar from vaginal incision into inner groin using a vaginal guide.

midline Prolene loop serves as a visual aid to help center the mesh. Both the loop and the lateral sutures are removed after the sling is tensioned to the surgeon's satisfaction (Figure 7-7; **Video 7-2**).

Outside-In Technique

1. Preoperative considerations, patient positioning, and anesthesia are similar to the inside-out technique.

2. The penetration site for the trocar is marked in the inner groin, which should be just below the adductor longus tendon, lateral to the clitoris (Figures 7-8 and 7-9). Placing an index finger in the vaginal fornix and the thumb in the inner groin facilitates appropriate location for needle penetration (see Figure 7-8).

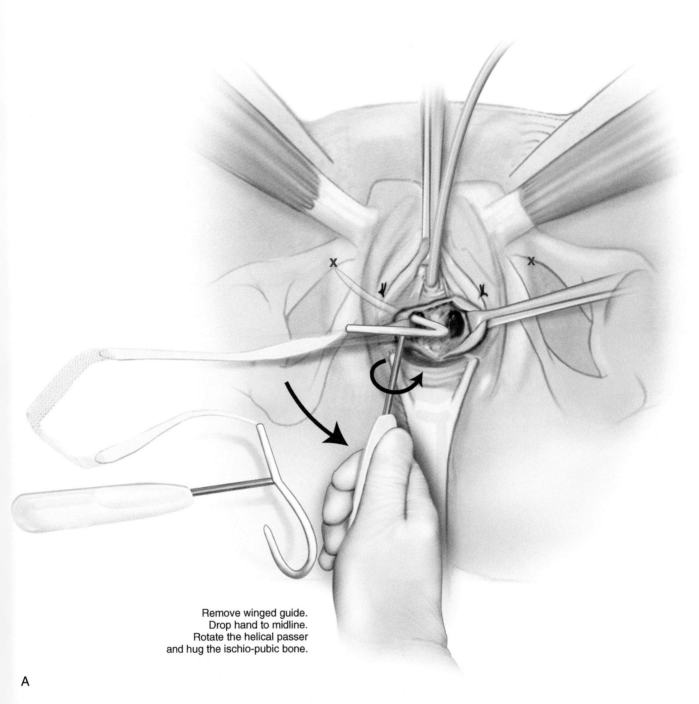

Remove winged guide.
Drop hand to midline.
Rotate the helical passer
and hug the ischio-pubic bone.

A

Figure 7-5 A, Technique of how to rotate inside-out TOT trocar handle through the obturator membrane and around the ischiopubic ramus.

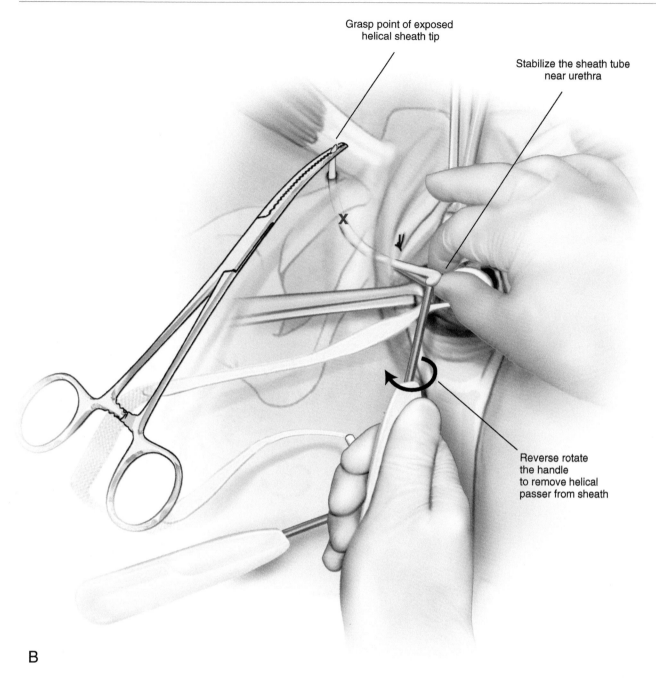

Grasp point of exposed
helical sheath tip

Stabilize the sheath tube
near urethra

X

Reverse rotate
the handle
to remove helical
passer from sheath

B

Figure 7-5, cont'd B, Technique of how best to remove helical trocar from sheath during inside-out technique for TOT sling.

3. *Vaginal incision.* The incision is similar to the inside-out technique.

4. *Vaginal dissection.* The dissection is carried laterally on both sides of the urethra aiming toward the obturator membrane. The incision should allow for the passage of the index finger to the level of the inferior pubic ramus (Figure 7-38).

5. *Trocar passage.* A stab wound is made with the scalpel at the previously marked puncture sites in the groin region, and the tip of the trocar is inserted into the stab wound. With the handle being nearly horizontal or parallel to the floor, the obturator membrane is penetrated, and the trocar handle is rotated and advanced along the ischiopubic ramus with the needle exiting into the vaginal space previously created. The initial rotation should

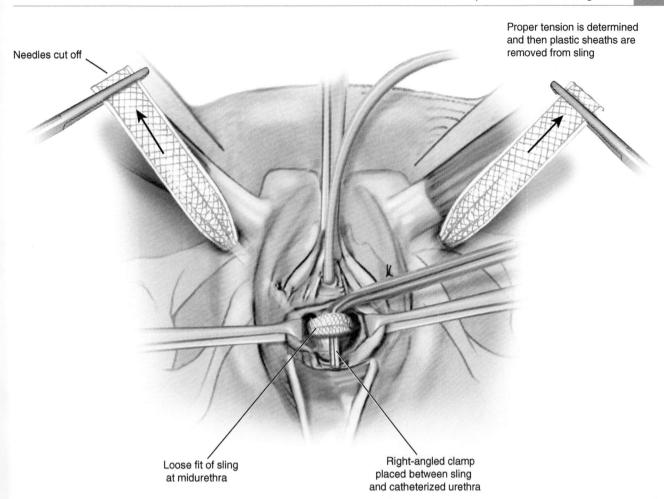

Needles cut off

Proper tension is determined
and then plastic sheaths are
removed from sling

Loose fit of sling
at midurethra

Right-angled clamp
placed between sling
and catheterized urethra

Figure 7-6 Technique of how best to tension inside-out TOT sling.

Figure 7-7 TVT-ABBREVO Sling
compared with conventional
TOT sling.

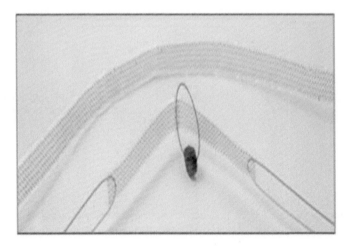

be to drop the handle of the trocar so that it becomes perpendicular to the floor. At the same time, the trocar handle is dropped from the initial near-horizontal starting position to the nearly vertical position; careful angling and "walking off" the bone allows for appropriate passage around the ischiopubic ramus (Figure 7-10).

6. *Cystoscopy*. Cystourethroscopy is performed as previously described for the inside-out technique.

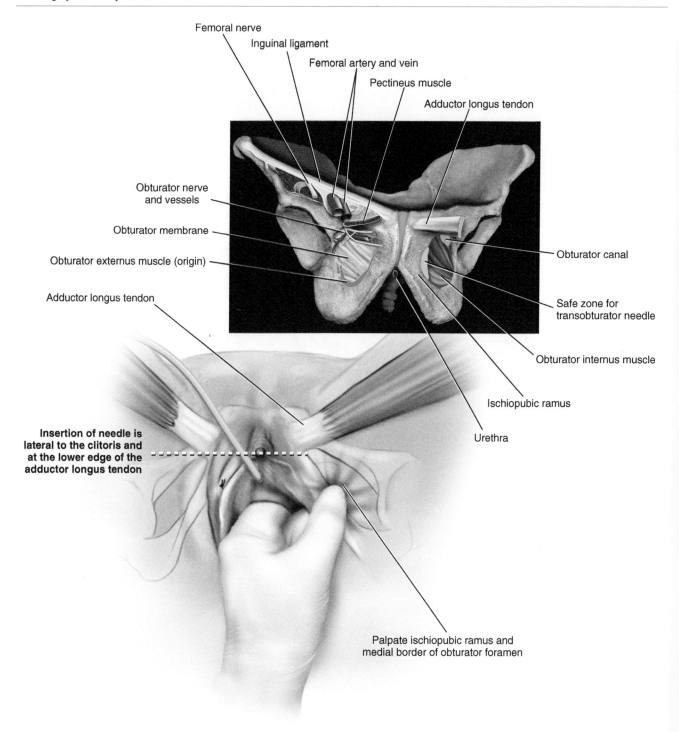

Femoral nerve

Inguinal ligament

Femoral artery and vein

Pectineus muscle

Adductor longus tendon

Obturator nerve and vessels

Obturator membrane

Obturator externus muscle (origin)

Adductor longus tendon

Obturator canal

Safe zone for transobturator needle

Obturator internus muscle

Ischiopubic ramus

Insertion of needle is lateral to the clitoris and at the lower edge of the adductor longus tendon

Urethra

Palpate ischiopubic ramus and medial border of obturator foramen

Figure 7-8 Penetration site for outside-in TOT. Trocar should be at the level of clitoris. which is just below the insertion of the adductor longus tendon. Placing an index finger in the anterior vaginal fornix and the thumb in the inner groin allows palpation of this location.

7. *Loading of the mesh.* The mesh is attached to the trocar and the needles are withdrawn, passing the sling and plastic sheath through the groin incision (Figure 7-11).

8. *Tensioning.* Tensioning is as described in the inside-out section, using a right-angled clamp (Figure 7-12).

9. The wound is irrigated, and the mucosal edges are approximated using a running 3-0 polyglycolic acid suture. The groin stab wounds are closed with absorbable suture or liquid tissue adhesive.

Figure 7-9 Anatomic location of clitoris and tendon of adductor longus. These are important landmarks when an outside-in TOT sling is being performed.

(From Baggish MS, Karram MM, eds. Atlas of Pelvic Anatomy and Gynecology Surgery, *ed 3. St. Louis: Saunders; 2011.)*

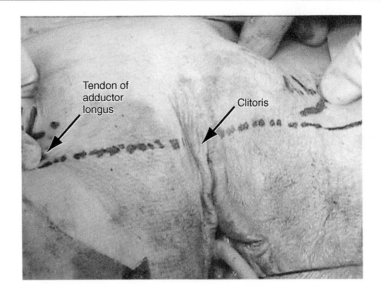

With thumb on curve of needle, push needle tip through skin incision until obturator membrane is perforated

Needle continues behind ischiopubic ramus

Rotate needle tip toward vaginal tunnel

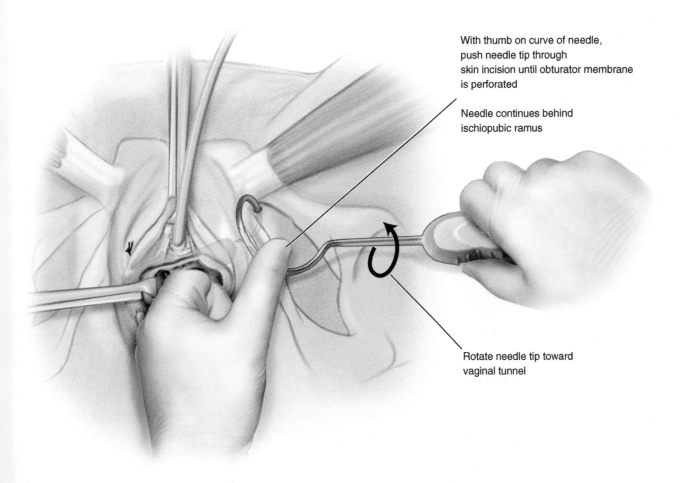

Figure 7-10 Technique for passage of outside-in trocar through the obturator membrane. Once the obturator membrane is penetrated, appropriate rotation of the handle is required for the needle to hug the back of the ischiopubic ramus.

Figure 7-11 After both outside-in needles are passed, the sling is attached to the needles. Cystoscopy is usually performed before pulling the sling through to the groin.

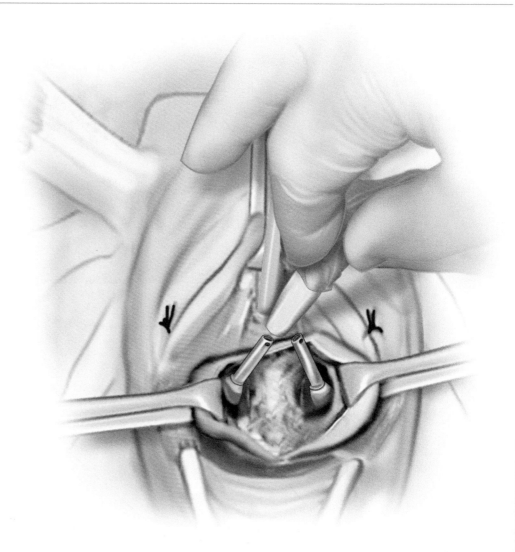

Connect mesh to needles on both sides

10. The catheter may be removed in the recovery room, and the patient is discharged after documenting voiding efficiency. If the patient is unable to void spontaneously, either intermittent self-catheterization is taught or the patient is discharged with an indwelling Foley catheter (**Video 7-3**).

Outcomes

A meta-analysis evaluating a phase II randomized controlled trial comparing retropubic and transobturator midurethral slings showed similar effectiveness in overall subjective outcomes. (Novara et al., 2010). A Cochrane review concluded that there was no subjective difference in cure rate or improvement between the two routes. This conclusion was based on 10 trials involving 1281 patients (Ogah et al., 2009). The same review reported a bladder perforation rate of 0.3% in the TOT group versus 5.5% in the retropubic group.

Outcomes of the two different placement techniques were evaluated in a meta-analysis by Latthe et al. (2010). No significant difference in subjective or objective SUI cure rates was observed. Also, there was no significant difference

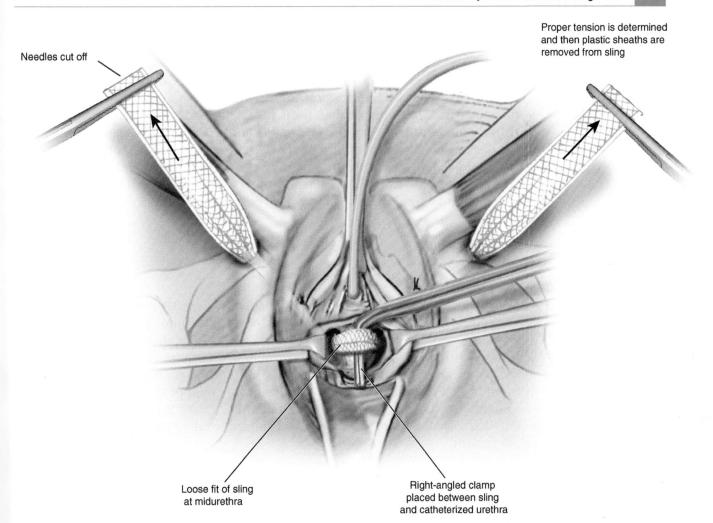

Needles cut off

Proper tension is determined and then plastic sheaths are removed from sling

Loose fit of sling at midurethra

Right-angled clamp placed between sling and catheterized urethra

Figure 7-12 Tension for outside-in TOT sling is identical to tension for inside-out TOT sling.

in the postoperative development of voiding difficulty or de novo urgency when the two techniques were compared. A randomized controlled trial by Abdel-Fattah et al. in 2010 also showed no difference in outcomes between the two techniques; however, when comparing these surgical approaches, the outside-in technique was associated with higher vaginal angle mucosal tears during placement.

In a retrospective study by Stav et al. (2010), ISD was shown to be an independent risk factor for unsuccessful outcomes with TOT slings with an odds ratio of 1.9 favoring retropubic slings. A similar study by Miller et al. (2006) showed higher success rates for retropubic slings versus TOT slings when the maximum urethral closure pressures were less than 40 mm Hg. Postoperative voiding dysfunction occurred less frequently in the TOT group (4% vs. 7% with relative risk 0.63) in this study.

Despite differences in technique and brand of mesh used, treatment success rates for uncomplicated primary SUI seem to be similar for the retropubic and TOT tension-free slings. The percentage of patients treated successfully ranges from 60% to 96% (depending on how "cure" is defined). When the definition of success is restricted to SUI symptoms, especially over a short time, the reported effectiveness is high. In contrast, when the definition of success includes incontinence of any type, the reported effectiveness is lower. In a study that reported 60% effectiveness, success was defined as no incontinence symptoms of any type, a negative cough stress test, and no subsequent retreatment for SUI or postoperative urinary retention. Retropubic slings, especially TVT, may be more effective for ISD, although this conclusion must be tempered by the small number of studies addressing the issue and differences in the diagnosis of ISD. Some studies have reported good success in treating mixed urinary incontinence with the retropubic and TOT sling, although other studies have reported that the initial benefit for urgency or urge incontinence is not sustained over time compared with the benefit for SUI. It is important to counsel patients before surgery that improvement in SUI symptoms and general satisfaction is highly likely, but perfect bladder function is not.

Complications

Voiding Dysfunction

Of women undergoing TOT sling procedures, 4% to 8% develop some form of voiding dysfunction. Initial postoperative management includes catheterization; however, if this persists, the option of sling lysis should be contemplated. Urethral dilation is typically not recommended because of fear of predisposing the patient to erosion of the sling material into the urethra. De novo development of urgency and urge incontinence occurs in approximately 6% of women undergoing TOT sling procedures (Ogah et al., 2009). See Chapter 9 for a more detailed discussion of how best to manage voiding dysfunction after sling placement.

Groin Pain

Groin pain is reported to occur in 16% of patients after TOT procedures. The inside-out technique seems to be associated with more groin pain compared with the outside-in technique. When postoperative groin pain occurs, it is usually deep within the tissue and manifests when the patient abducts or adducts her legs. This pain is reported to be less common in patients who are overweight (body mass index >30). The motivation for development of the newer TVT-Abbrevo sling was to prevent postoperative groin pain by not having any sling material present in the inner groin muscles. In almost all cases the pain is self-limited. In situations in which it is more severe or persistent, local injections of a long-acting anesthetic in combination with a steroid may be attempted.

Dyspareunia

Dyspareunia has been reported to occur in 9% of patients. A randomized controlled trial by Ross et al. (2009) mentioned the concerning fact that the sling tape may be frequently palpable postoperatively in patients with TOT slings. In addition to the risk for dyspareunia, palpable sling tape may predispose to erosions. Excision of the palpable portion of the sling is usually curative of the dyspareunia but may predispose the patient to a recurrence of her SUI.

Vaginal Mesh Erosion

Vaginal mesh erosion is a known complication associated with all types of synthetic slings. It occurs in up to 7% of women who have undergone a TOT sling procedure. Based on symptomatology and the size and location of the erosion, appropriate management steps should be taken. These could involve simple observation in the asymptomatic patient vs. local estrogen cream vs. attempts at mobilization of healthy vaginal wall over the eroded tape vs. complete excision of the eroded tape.

Conclusion

With appropriate patient selection and placement, TOT slings have been shown to be very successful procedures for the correction of SUI.

Suggested Readings

Abdel-Fattah M, Ramsay I, Pringle S, et al. Randomised prospective single-blinded study comparing "inside-out" versus "outside-in" transobturator tapes in the management of urodynamic stress incontinence: 1-year outcomes from the E-TOT study. *BJOG*. 2010;117:870-878.

Abdel-Fattah M, et al. Evaluation of transobturator tension-free vaginal tapes in the management of women with mixed urinary incontinence: one-year outcomes. *Am J Obstet Gynecol*. 2011;205: 150.e1-150.e6.

American College of Obstetricians and Gynecologists. Urinary incontinence in women. ACOG Practice Bulletin No. 63. *Obstet Gynecol*. 2005;105:1533-1545.

Barber MD, Kleeman S, Karram MM, et al. Transobturator tape compared with tension-free vaginal tape for the treatment of stress urinary incontinence: a randomized controlled trial. *Obstet Gynecol*. 2008;111:611-621.

Brubaker L, Cundiff GW, Fine P, et al. Pelvic Floor Disorders Network. Abdominal sacrocolpopexy with Burch colposuspension to reduce urinary stress incontinence. *N Engl J Med*. 2006;354:1557-1566.

But I, Faganelj M. Complications and short-term results of two different transobturator techniques for surgical treatment of women with urinary incontinence: a randomized study. *Int Urogynecol J*. 2008;19:857-861.

Cadish LA, Hacker MR, Dodge LE, Dramitinos P, Hota LS, Elkadry EA. Association of body mass index with hip and thigh pain following transobturator midurethral sling placement. *Am J Obstet Gynecol*. 2010;203:508.e1-508.e5.

Deffieux X, Daher N, Mansoor A, Debodinance P, Muhlstein J, Fernandez H. Transobturator TVT-O versus retropubic TVT: results of a multicenter randomized controlled trial at 24 months follow-up. *Int Urogynecol J*. 2010;21:1337-1345.

Delorme E. Transobturator urethral suspension: mini-invasive procedure in the treatment of stress urinary incontinence in women. *Prog Urol*. 2001;11(6):1306-1313.

Kaelin-Gambirasio I, Jacob S, Boulvain M, Dubuisson JB, Dällenbach P. Complications associated with transobturator sling procedures: analysis of 233 consecutive cases with a 27 months follow-up. *BMC Womens Health*. 2009;9:28.

Latthe PM, Singh P, Foon R, Toozs-Hobson P. Two routes of transobturator tape procedures in stress urinary incontinence: a meta-analysis with direct and indirect comparison of randomized trials. *BJU Int*. 2010;106:68-76.

Liapis A, Bakas P, Creatsas G. Monarc vs TVT-O for the treatment of primary stress incontinence: a randomized study. *Int Urogynecol J*. 2008;19:185-190.

Meschia M, Bertozzi R, Pifarotti P, et al. Perioperative morbidity and early results of a randomised trial comparing TVT and TVT-O. *Int Urogynecol J*. 2007;18:1257-1261.

Miller JJ, Botros SM, Akl MN, et al. Is transobturator tape as effective as tension-free vaginal tape in patients with borderline maximum urethral closure pressure? *Am J Obstet Gynecol*. 2006;195: 1799-1804.

Neuman M. TVT-obturator: short-term data on an operative procedure for the cure of female stress urinary incontinence performed on 300 patients. *Eur Urol*. 2007;51:1083-1087; discussion 1088.

Novara G, Artibani W, Barber MD, et al. Updated systematic review and meta-analysis of the comparative date on colposuspension, pubovaginal slings, and midurethral tapes in the surgical treatment of female stress urinary incontinence. *Eur Urol*. 2010;58:218-238.

Ogah J, Cody JD, Rogerson L. Minimally invasive synthetic suburethral sling operations for stress urinary incontinence in women. *Cochrane Database Syst Rev*. 2009;(4):CD006375.

Reyna JA, Terry PJ. Transobturator versus transabdominal mid urethral slings: a multi-institutional comparison of obstructive voiding complications. *J Urol*. 2006;175(3 Pt 1):1014-1017.

Richter HE, Albo ME, Zyczynski HM, et al. Urinary Incontinence Treatment Network. Retropubic versus transobturator midurethral slings for stress incontinence. *N Engl J Med.* 2010;362: 2066-2076.

Ross S, Robert M, Swaby C, et al. Transobturator tape compared with tension-free vaginal tape for stress incontinence: a randomized controlled trial. *Obstet Gynecol.* 2009;114:1287-1294.

Scheiner DA, Betschart C, Wiederkehr S, Seifert B, Fink D, Perucchini D. Twelve months effect on voiding function of retropubic compared with outside-in and inside-out transobturator midurethral slings. *Int Urogynecol J.* 2012;23:197-206.

Schierlitz L, Dwyer PL, Rosamilia A, et al. Three-year follow-up of tension-free vaginal tape compared with transobturator tape in women with stress urinary incontinence and intrinsic sphincter deficiency. *Obstet Gynecol.* 2012;119(2 Pt 1):321-327.

Sentilhes L, Berthier A, Loisel C, Descamps P, Marpeau L, Grise P. Female sexual function following surgery for stress urinary incontinence: tension-free vaginal versus transobturator tape procedure. *Int Urogynecol J.* 2009;20:393-399.

Stav K, Dwyer PL, Rosamilia A, Schierlitz L, Lim YN, Lee J. Risk factors of treatment failure of midurethral sling procedures for women with urinary stress incontinence. *Int Urogynecol J.* 2010; 21:149-155.

Sung VW, Schleinitz MD, Rardin CR, Ward RM, Myers DL. Comparison of retropubic vs transobturator approach to midurethral slings: a systematic review and meta-analysis. *Am J Obstet Gynecol.* 2007;197:3-11.

Wei J. Pelvic Floor Disorders Network. The value of the preoperative prolapse reduction stress test in women without stress incontinence symptoms undergoing vaginal prolapse surgery with or without TVT: results from the OPUS trial. *Female Pelvic Med Reconstr Surg.* 2001;17(5 Suppl 2):S53.

Yoshizawa T, Yamaguchi K, Obinata D, Sato K, Mochida J, Takahashi S. Laparoscopic transvesical removal of erosive mesh after transobturator tape procedure. *Int J Urol.* 2011;18:861-863.

Zahn CM, Siddique S, Hernandez S, Lockrow EG. Anatomic comparison of two transobturator tape procedures. *Obstet Gynecol.* 2007;109:701-706.

Single-Incision Synthetic Midurethral Slings

Mickey Karram, M.D.
W. Stuart Reynolds, M.D.
Dani Zoorob, M.D.
Roger Dmochowski, M.D.

 Videos

8-1 TVT-Secur—Hammock Placement
8-2 TVT-Secur—"U" Placement
8-3 MiniArc Single-Incision Sling System

8-4 Solyx SIS System
8-5 AJUST Adjustable Single-Incision Sling

Introduction

In 2006, the single-incision synthetic midurethral sling was introduced as a modification to traditional retropubic and transobturator midurethral slings (MUS). These slings were designed to require less dissection in the midurethral area without the need to make additional incisions suprapubically or in the groin. They are placed entirely through an incision in the vagina having no exit point. They were designed to minimize the risk of bladder perforation associated with traditional retropubic MUS and the risk of groin discomfort or other issues related to the inner thigh associated with passage of transobturator slings through the obturator membrane and adductor compartment. Single-incision minislings are anchored into the obturator internus muscle or connective tissue of the endopelvic fascia of the retropubic space behind the pubic bone, depending on the configuration of the sling chosen by the surgeon. A survey of urologists in the United States suggests that 10% of practicing urologists have already adopted this technology for regular use in patients with primary stress urinary incontinence (SUI). However, the U.S. Food and Drug Administration (FDA) has required the manufacturers of single-incision slings to pursue additional studies to document long-term efficacy and safety further. These studies, which will be ongoing over the next 2 years, will determine the future of these devices.

Indications and Patient Selection

Indications for the single-incision slings are similar to the indications for the more traditional MUS. Because these slings are less invasive than a retropubic or transobturator MUS, they may be desirous for some special patient populations. Because they avoid the retropubic space, the minisling may be considered specifically in patients who have undergone previous retropubic and abdominal procedures and may be at higher risk for significant pelvic adhesions. Because it does not entail complete passage of trocars to the skin level, it may be considered in patients with significant soft tissue mass or obesity in the areas of tradition MUS trocar site exit (i.e., truncal or intertrigonal obesity) that may surpass the length of the trocar. Because single-incision minisling procedures can be done under local anesthesia, they can also be considered in patients with significant comorbidities in whom general anesthesia is contraindicated. At the present time, the authors rarely use single-incision slings in patients with primary SUI because long-term data showing efficacy comparable to retropubic or transobturator MUS are lacking (see Outcomes section).

Description of Various Types of Single-Incision Slings

Five single-incision minislings are commercially available at the present time in the United States: TVT-Secur (Ethicon Women's Health & Urology, Somerville, NJ), MiniArc Single-Incision Sling system (American Medical Systems, Minnetonka, MN), Solyx SIS system (Boston Scientific Corp, Natick, MA), AJUST Adjustable Single-Incision Sling (Bard, Covington, GA), and Minitape (MPathy Medical, Raynham, MA).

The TVT-Secur is a preassembled polypropylene (Prolene) woven mesh tape (8 cm × 1.1 cm) and metal inserter device. Sandwiching each end of the tape are polyglactin-910 (Vicryl) and polydioxanone (PDS) woven fleece patches that are designed to allow connective tissue ingrowth while undergoing concurrent absorption (within 90 to 180 days) encouraging the permanent fixation of the mesh sling. The sling and inserter device are inserted and the position of the sling is confirmed, after which the inserter device is disengaged and removed, leaving the mesh behind.

The MiniArc Single-Incision Sling (Figure 8-1) is a polypropylene mesh (8.5 cm × 1.1 cm) with permanent self-fixating tips that is deployed with a supplied metal 2.3-mm needle/trocar. The mesh is connected to the tip of the

Figure 8-1 MiniArc Single-Incision Sling.

(Courtesy American Medical Systems, Minnetonka, MN.)

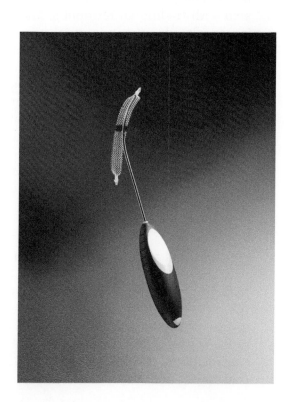

needle before insertion; the mesh and needle are inserted; and the needle is removed, leaving the mesh behind. Self-fixating tips are constructed of polypropylene and have two anchoring barbs that help resist up to 5.5 lb of pull-out force to remove the mesh. A redocking maneuver can be set up before insertion to allow retrieval and reinsertion of the mesh if necessary.

The Solyx SIS system (Boston Scientific Corp., Natick, MA; Figure 8-2) includes a polypropylene mesh tape (9 cm in length) with permanent barbed self-fixating tips and a metal and plastic delivery device or trocar. This system is designed similarly to the MiniArc Single-Incision Sling system, in that each tip of the sling is sequentially attached to the end of the delivery device for mesh placement, which is removed after insertion. The edges of the center 4 cm of the mesh (advertised as the suburethral portion) are bonded together to potentially reduce irritation and the possibility of mesh erosion or extrusion.

The AJUST Adjustable Single-Incision Sling (Bard Medical, Covington, GA; Figure 8-3) is a new adjustable minisling that allows the surgeon to tighten or loosen the sling after it has been anchored into the obturator membrane.

Case 1: Stress Incontinence in a Patient with Significant Co-Morbidities

A 64-year-old, morbidly obese (body mass index 44) woman presents with symptoms of severe SUI. She has a history of significant cardiac disease. She desires definitive therapy for SUI. Cardiac clearance is obtained for the patient to have a procedure under local anesthesia with intravenous sedation. The patient undergoes a single-incision sling procedure under local anesthesia. During the procedure, a cough stress test is used to guide how tightly to place the sling. The surgery is done as an outpatient procedure, and the patient is discharged without a catheter.

Discussion of Case

In this case, a single-incision sling was chosen because the procedure could be done under minimal anesthesia, and the tensioning of a single-incision sling is more straightforward when using a cough stress test. With retropubic or transobturator MUS, when an intraoperative cough stress test is used to tension the sling, the patient should still leak a small amount of urine, which is a very subjective endpoint. A single-incision sling can be tensioned to the point of continence at the time of surgery with very little chance of retention or voiding dysfunction, which is a more objective endpoint.

Surgical Techniques

Figure 8-4 illustrates how the authors prefer to tension various synthetic MUS.

TVT-Secur

1. *Preoperative considerations.* Insertion of a minisling may be performed under many different types of anesthesia, including general, spinal or epidural, regional, and local. Perioperative antibiotics (e.g., fluoroquinolone or first-generation cephalosporin) are generally administered before the incision.

2. *Patient positioning.* The patient is positioned in the dorsal lithotomy position with legs in stirrups. The perineum and vagina are sterilely prepared and draped so as to exclude the anus. Lateral labia majora retraction stitches may be placed or a self-retaining retractor may be used to improve vaginal exposure. A weighted vaginal speculum is placed, and bladder drainage is accomplished with a Foley catheter.

Figure 8-2 Solyx SIS.

(Courtesy Boston Scientific Corp, Natick, MA.)

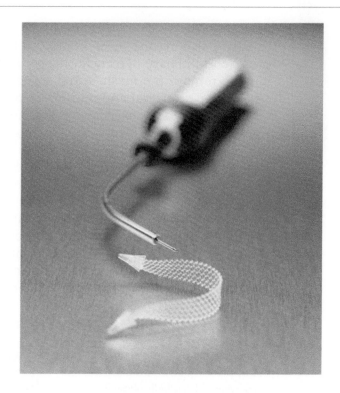

Figure 8-3 AJUST Adjustable Single-Incision Sling.

(Bard Medical, Covington, GA.)

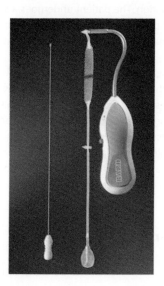

3. *Vaginal incision.* A 1- to 1.5-cm midline incision is marked starting 1 cm below the urethral meatus, and the area is infiltrated with injectable grade saline or 1% lidocaine with epinephrine for hydrodissection of the periurethral tissues. An Allis clamp may be placed distal to the incision, with care taken not to traumatize the urethral meatus, to facilitate visualization. An incision is made sharply with a scalpel.

4. *Vaginal flap dissection.* Dissection of lateral vaginal flaps proceeds in a standard fashion with attention to developing an appropriately robust and well-vascularized vaginal flap, while not jeopardizing the thickness of the periurethral tissue. This flap is carried laterally and anteriorly until the

Figure 8-4 Tensioning of synthetic midurethral slings. **A,** Synthetic retropubic slings are usually left very loose, easily allowing an instrument to be passed between the sling and the posterior urethra. **B,** Transobturator synthetic midurethral slings are usually tensioned slightly tighter than retropubic slings. **C,** Single-incision slings are tensioned so that they come in direct contact with the posterior urethra, making it very difficult to pass an instrument between the sling and the posterior urethra.

(From Baggish MS, Karram MM, eds. Atlas of Pelvic Anatomy and Gynecology Surgery, *ed 3. St. Louis: Saunders; 2011.)*

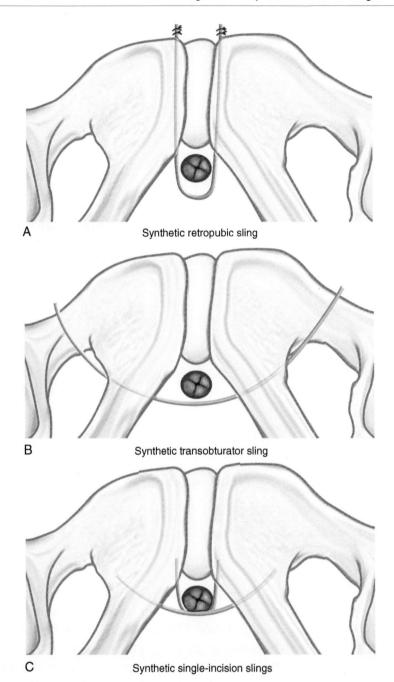

A   Synthetic retropubic sling

B   Synthetic transobturator sling

C   Synthetic single-incision slings

endopelvic fascia is encountered, but the retropubic space is not entered (Figure 8-5).

5. *Preparation of sling (TVT-Secur).* The sling is prepared by soaking in saline mixed with antibiotic (e.g., cephalexin). When ready to use, a stout, medium-length needle driver is attached to one of the metal arms of the device. This driver is used to assist in placement and to protect the disengagement pin.

6. *Configuration of sling placement.* The sling may be placed in either of two angle configurations that mimic the angles of support achieved by either a transobturator or retropubic MUS. Inserting the device at a 90-degree angle to the sagittal midline achieves the angle of support similar to a transobturator sling, or what has been termed the "hammock" configuration.

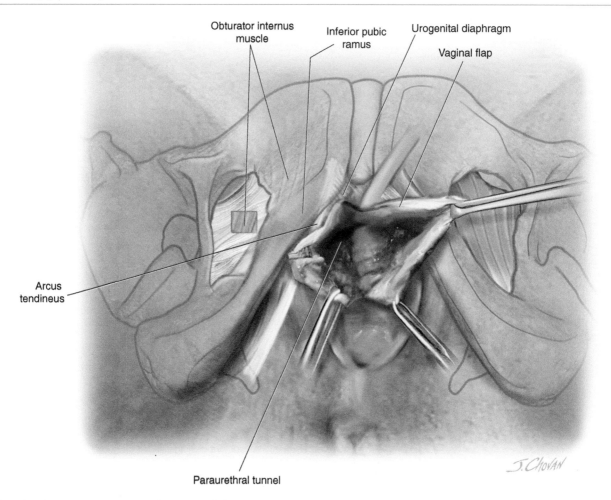

Obturator internus muscle

Inferior pubic ramus

Urogenital diaphragm

Vaginal flap

Arcus tendineus

Paraurethral tunnel

J. Chovan

Figure 8-5 Appropriate anterior vaginal incision made for a single-incision sling. Dissection extends paraurethrally to inferior pubic ramus.

(From Baggish MS, Karram MM, eds. Atlas of Pelvic Anatomy and Gynecology Surgery, *ed 3. St. Louis: Saunders; 2011.)*

Angling at 45 degrees from the sagittal midline achieves the angle of support similar to the retropubic sling, or what has been termed the "U" configuration (Figure 8-6; **Videos 8-1** and **8-2**).

7. *Insertion of sling.* To place the TVT-Secur, the tip of the inserter (without the protective cap) is positioned in the previously dissected periurethral space, angling toward the ipsilateral shoulder for the "U" configuration or toward the 9 o'clock or 3 o'clock position for the hammock configuration, and gently inserted until resistance from the pubic bone is met (no more than 3 to 4 cm). The inserter is slightly withdrawn, angled more posteriorly, and reinserted to "walk off" the pubic bone. When the posterior edge of the bone is encountered (noted by a loss of resistance), the inserter is gently driven along the posterior surface of the bone into the connective tissue of the urogenital diaphragm. Maintaining close contact with the posterior surface of the pubic bone minimizes chance of injury to pelvic structures; this is facilitated by rotating the device as it is advanced with the index finger applying pressure on the finger pad of the inserter arm and lowering the needle driver toward the floor. When the inserter is firmly embedded in the connective tissue, insertion is stopped, the needle driver is removed and replaced to the contralateral inserter arm, and the maneuver is repeated on the contralateral side.

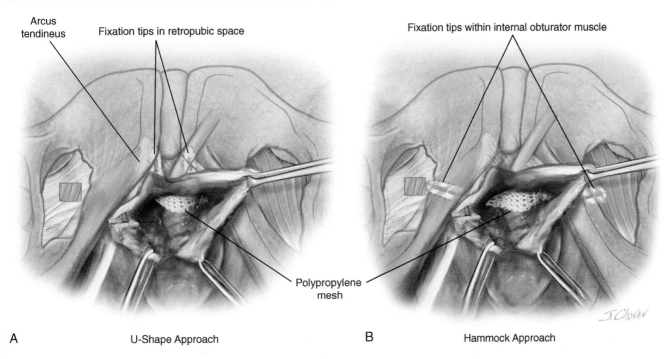

Arcus tendineus

Fixation tips in retropubic space

Fixation tips within internal obturator muscle

Polypropylene mesh

A   U-Shape Approach

B   Hammock Approach

J. Chovan

Figure 8-6 Technique for TVT-Secur placement demonstrating both "U" **(A)** and hammock **(B)** placement.

8. *Cystoscopy.* Cystoscopy is performed to evaluate for bladder injury. The bladder must be completely filled and examined in its entirety with a 30-degree or 70-degree lens or both. If a trocar injury occurs, it is typically located at the posterior lateral aspect of the bladder base. Gently wiggling the inserter arms under cystoscopic guidance shows their location relative to the bladder mucosa.

9. *Tensioning.* The tension of the sling may be assessed by gently inserting an angled clamp between the mesh and the urethra. An appropriate amount of tension in the sling permits just the insertion of the tip of the clamp but not more. If the sling is deemed either too loose or too tight, it can either be inserted further or can be gently retracted, always by moving the inserter arm and not the mesh directly.

10. *Deploying and disengaging blade.* To deploy the mesh sling and disengage the inserter arm, the release wire is pulled to the stop position while stabilizing the inserter; the inserter is withdrawn with a gentle twisting motion. This is repeated for the other side.

11. *Vaginal closure.* The vaginal incision is closed with a No. 2-0 absorbable running suture. A bladder catheter and vaginal packing are placed temporarily and removed in the recovery room when the patient is awake. A voiding trial can immediately be performed.

MiniArc and Solyx Single-Incision Sling

1. Placement of both the MiniArc and Solyx minislings proceeds by the same initial steps as outlined previously (steps 1-4). The direction of dissection is aimed at a 45-degree angle to the midline, toward the location of the insertion of the adductor longus tendon on the pubic ramus.

2. *Preparation of the sling.* The sling is prepared by inserting the tip of the delivery device or needle into the self-affixing end of the mesh apparatus,

ensuring that the mesh is orientated on the outside of bend of the delivery needle.

3. *Insertion of sling.* To place the MiniArc or Solyx minislings, the tip of the delivery needle with mesh assembly attached is inserted into the previously dissected vaginal space and aimed along a path 45 degrees from the midline. Placement should be immediately posterior to the ischiopubic ramus; the needle can be "walked off" the posterior aspect of the bone as described previously, maintaining a close proximity to the posterior surface of the bone. The tip should be advanced until the midline marking on the mesh is situated under the middle of the urethra. The needle is removed from the mesh, attached to the other end of the mesh device, and inserted on the contralateral side in a similar manner, ensuring the mesh lies flat under the urethra, until the proper degree of desired tension is achieved. The delivery device is disengaged and removed (Figures 8-7 and 8-8). The MiniArc

Figure 8-7 Technique for placement of the MiniArc Single-Incision Sling. The sling is placed directly into the obturator internus muscle.

(From Baggish MS, Karram MM, eds. Atlas of Pelvic Anatomy and Gynecology Surgery, *ed 3. St. Louis: Saunders; 2011.)*

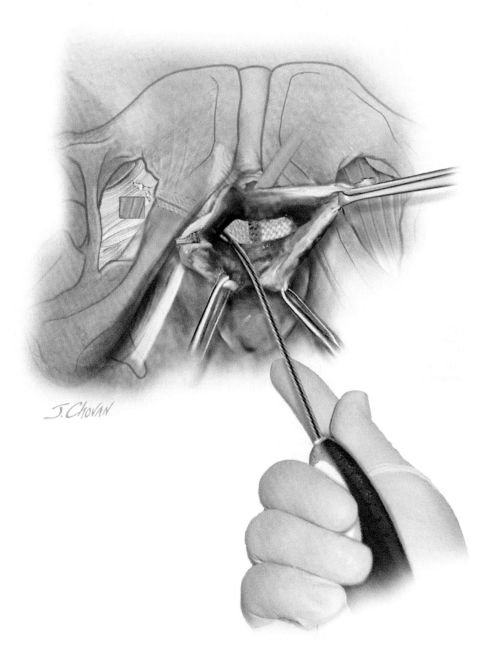

Single-Incision Sling can be arranged with a delivery/inserter needle to facilitate reconnecting the needle tip into the self-affixing tip of the mesh device. This arrangement allows for the mesh to be inserted further, if more tension is desired. The redocking procedure entails threading a 2-0 polypropylene suture through the tip of the mesh assembly and then through the tip of the delivery device, knotting one end. This end of the mesh is placed first, in the usual fashion, then the delivery needle is removed, leaving the suture in place. The opposite side is also placed as previously described. If further tensioning is warranted, the free end of the suture is reinserted into the end of the delivery needle, and the needle is advanced along the suture, sliding into the tip of the mesh device. Once docked, the entire mesh device can be advanced further into the patient.

4. *Cystoscopy.* Cystoscopy should be performed to evaluate for bladder injury.

5. *Vaginal closure.* The vaginal incision is closed in the same way as described previously (**Videos 8-3** and **8-4**).

Figure 8-8 Placement of the Solyx SIS.

(Courtesy Boston Scientific Corp, Natick, MA.)

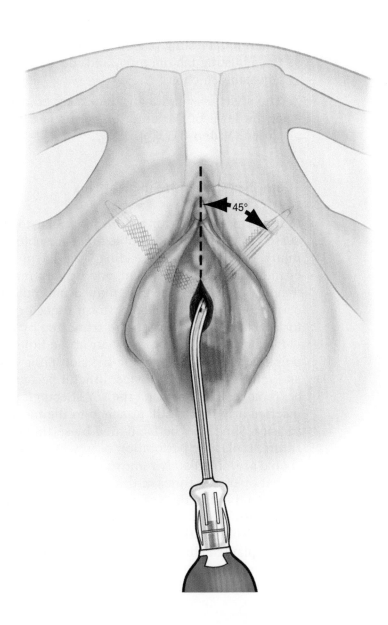

AJUST Adjustable Single-Incision Sling

1. Placement of the AJUST Adjustable Single-Incision Sling proceeds by the same initial steps (steps 1-4) as previously outlined.

2. After appropriate dissection is completed, the fixed anchor is pushed into the tissue until it is slightly beyond the ischiopubic ramus. The handle is pivoted toward the obturator internus muscle and membrane. The fixed anchor is pushed through the obturator internus muscle and membrane. It should be ensured that the midline indicator is at or slightly past the midurethra in the direction of insertion.

3. The fixed anchor is released by pushing the anchor release lever forward, and the introducer is removed. Gentle traction is applied to the suburethral sling to confirm proper fixation.

4. The adjustable anchor is loaded into the introducer and secured by retracting the anchor release lever. Steps 1 through 3 are repeated on the contralateral side.

5. The adjustable anchor is stabilized at its insertion point while gently pulling on the adjustment tab, and the sling is adjusted. To loosen the sling, gentle countertraction is applied to the suburethral sling on the adjustable side of the sling implant.

6. When proper sling placement is achieved, the flexible stylet is inserted into the adjusting tab opening, and the sling lock is pushed into place up to the adjustable anchor.

7. The stylet is withdrawn, the excess adjustment mesh lateral to the urethra at the level of the anterior sulcus is trimmed, and the vaginal incision is closed (**Video 8-5**).

Complications and Surgical Tips

Complications that can occur are similar to the complications previously discussed in regard to retropubic and transobturator MUS. These include bladder injury or perforation, bleeding, vaginal mesh extrusion, urinary tract mesh erosion, voiding dysfunction, and urinary retention. Viscous organ damage and major vascular injury still may occur but in theory should be much less common because the needle/trocar trajectory through the retropubic or obturator space is significantly more truncated by design of the minisling.

Bladder perforation may occur at the time of sling insertion; the self-affixing points of the MiniArc Single-Incision Sling and Solyx SIS may make removal and reinsertion of the device difficult because these slings are not designed to be removed. Removal of the TVT-Secur is accomplished by pulling out the inserted arm that is still attached to the mesh. Removal of the MiniArc Single-Incision Sling may be facilitated by setting up the redocking procedure with a suture. If bladder perforation occurs and is discovered on cystoscopy, the sling should be immediately removed. A secondary insertion should not be attempted at that operative time. In the authors' opinion, cystoscopy should be routinely performed at the time of placement of a single-incision sling.

Because of the shorter length of inserted mesh, more tension is placed on the minisling at the time of insertion than is placed on other types of MUS. The implanted sling should be in close apposition to the urethra with no laxity in the material. The surgeon should use a clamp or right angle to determine that there is no redundancy in the sling material.

Outcomes

Compared with transobturator and retropubic slings, long-term outcomes of single-incision slings vary depending on the study. Barber et al. (2012), De Ridder et al. (2010), and Neuman et al. (2011) showed similar cure rates when compared to retropubic or transobturator MUS, whereas Wang et al. (2011) and Hinoul et al. (2011) showed higher long-term curerates for retropubic or transobturator MUS. The randomized controlled trial by Hinoul et al. (2011) involved 160 patients; the randomized controlled trial by Wang et al. (2011) comprised 106 patients. The randomized controlledtrial by Barber et al. (2012) involved 263 patients, the retrospective study by De Ridder et al. (2010) comprised 131 patients, and the prospective nonrandomized study by Neuman et al. (2011) contained 146 patients. A meta-analysis by Abdel-Fattah et al. in 2011 involving 758 women showed inferior subjective and objective cure rates over 6-month and 12-month periods for single-incision slings relative to transobturator and retropubic slings. The need for repeat incontinence surgery for patients with prior single-incision slings was significantly greater (relative risk, 6.72; confidence interval, 2.39-18.89), and there was increased de novo urgency (relative risk, 2.08; confidence interval, 1.01-4.28). The study by Abdel-Fattah et al. (2011) found that single-incision slings were associated with shorter operative times and lower pain scores immediately postoperatively.

Conclusion

At the present time, the future of single-incision slings is questionable because the FDA has required the manufacturers of these kits to pursue further studies to evaluate efficacy and safety. If the data eventually demonstrate acceptable long-term durability and safety, increased popularity is likely owing to the minimal invasiveness of these procedures.

Suggested Readings

Abdel-Fattah M, Ford JA, Lim CP, Madhuvrata P. Single-incision mini-slings versus standard midurethral slings in surgical management of female stress urinary incontinence: a meta-analysis of effectiveness and complications. *Eur Urol.* 2011;60:468-480.

Anger JT, Weinberg AE, Albo ME, et al. Trends in surgical management of stress urinary incontinence among female Medicare beneficiaries. *Urology.* 2009;74:283-287.

Barber MD, Weidner AC, Sokol AI, et al; Foundation for Female Health Awareness Research Network. Single-incision mini-sling compared with tension-free vaginal tape for the treatment of stress urinary incontinence: a randomized controlled trial. *Obstet Gynecol.* 2012;119(2 Pt 1):328-337.

Basu M, Duckett J. A randomised trial of a retropubic tension-free vaginal tape versus a mini-sling for stress incontinence. *BJOG.* 2010;117:730-735.

Cornu JN, Sebe P, Peyrat L, Ciofu C, Cussenot O, Haab F. Midterm prospective evaluation of TVT-Secur reveals high failure rate. *Eur Urol.* 2010;58:157-161.

De Ridder D, Berkers J, Deprest J, et al. Single incision mini-sling versus a transobutaror sling: a comparative study on MiniArc and Monarc slings. *Int Urogynecol J.* 2010;21:773-778.

Gauruder-Burmester A, Popken G. The MiniArc sling system in the treatment of female stress urinary incontinence. *Int Braz J Urol.* 2009;35:334-341.

Hinoul P, Vervest HA, den Boon J, et al. A randomized, controlled trial comparing an innovative single incision sling with an established transobturator sling to treat female stress urinary incontinence. *J Urol.* 2011;185:1356-1362.

Meschia M, Barbacini P, Baccichet R, et al. Short term outcomes with the Ajust system: a new single incision sling for the treatment of stress urinary incontinence. *Int Urogynecol J.* 2011;22:177-182.

Minassian VA, Stewart WF, Wood GC. Urinary incontinence in women: variation in prevalence estimates and risk factors. *Obstet Gynecol.* 2008;111(2 Pt 1):324-331.

Molden SM, Lucente VR. New minimally invasive slings: TVT Secur. *Curr Urol Rep.* 2008;9:358-361.

Moore RD, Mitchell GK, Miklos JR. Single-center retrospective study of the technique, safety, and 12-month efficacy of the MiniArc single-incision sling: a new minimally invasive procedure for treatment of female SUI. *Surg Technol Int.* 2009;18:175-181.

Neuman M, Sosnovski V, Kais M, Ophir E, Bornstein J. Transobturator vs single-incision suburethral mini-slings for treatment of female stress urinary incontinence: early postoperative pain and 3-year follow-up. *J Minim Invasive Gynecol.* 2011;18:769-773.

North CE, Hilton P, Ali-Ross NS, Smith AR. A 2-year observational study to determine the efficacy of a novel single incision sling procedure (Minitape) for female stress urinary incontinence. *BJOG.* 2010;117:356-360.

Serels S, Douso M, Short G. Preliminary findings with the Solyx single-incision sling system in female stress urinary incontinence. *Int Urogynecol J.* 2010;21:557-561.

Thom DH, Nygaard IE, Calhoun EA. Urologic diseases in America project: urinary incontinence in women—national trends in hospitalizations, office visits, treatment and economic impact. *J Urol.* 2005;173:1295-1301.

Walsh CA. TVT-Secur mini-sling for stress urinary incontinence: a review of outcomes at 12 months. *BJU Int.* 2011;108:652-657.

Wang YJ, Li FP, Wang Q, Yang S, Cai XG, Chen YH. Comparison of three mid-urethral tension-free tapes (TVT, TVT-O, and TVT-Secur) in the treatment of female stress urinary incontinence: 1-year follow-up. *Int Urogynecol J.* 2011;22:1369-1374.

Surgical Management of Voiding Dysfunction and Retention After Stress Incontinence Surgery

9

Mickey Karram, M.D.
Roger Dmochowski, M.D.

 Videos

9-1 Loosening of Retropubic Synthetic Sling at 8 Days Postoperatively
9-2 Excision of Suburethral Portion of Retropubic Synthetic Sling
9-3 Excision of Single-Incision Synthetic Sling

9-4 Incision of Pubovaginal Sling
9-5 Retropubic Vesicourethrolysis
9-6 Vaginal Urethrolysis

Introduction

The true incidence of voiding dysfunction and iatrogenic obstruction after anti-incontinence surgery is unknown and likely underestimated because of underdiagnosis, misdiagnosis, variations in definition, and underreporting. Reported rates of obstruction vary depending on the type of anti-incontinence surgery performed. Urinary obstruction requiring intervention after any anti-incontinence surgery occurs in at least 1% to 2% of patients even in the hands of the most experienced surgeon.

Voiding dysfunction after surgery for stress urinary incontinence (SUI) can be related to various degrees of obvious outlet obstruction, de novo development of detrusor overactivity, or a significant worsening of pre-existing detrusor overactivity. Historically, textbooks have also discussed the potential for impaired contractility to be a cause in such situations. When patients present with various degrees of voiding dysfunction or symptomatic overactive bladder symptoms, the surgeon must go to great lengths to construct a management plan to address these very distressing symptoms.

Patients with iatrogenic obstruction or voiding dysfunction after surgery for SUI can present with many symptoms. The most obvious signs and symptoms include complete or partial urinary retention, inability to void continuously, and the presence of a slow stream with a prolonged voiding time with or without intermittency. Also, many women with milder forms of outlet obstruction complain of having to lean back or even stand up to void. Some women do not have obstructive voiding symptoms and present mainly with the de novo

Table 9–1 Reported rates of obstruction from various sling procedures

	TVT	Transobturator Tape (Outside-In)	TVT-O (Inside-Out)	TVT-Secur	Pubovaginal Sling	SPARC	Retropubic Suspension	Transvaginal Needle Suspension
Urinary retention (including transient obstruction that may not be clinically relevant)	0-43%	0-7.8%	0-10.3%	2%-8%	2%-47%	0-18.1%	3%-7%	4%-8%
Retention requiring CIC >1 wk	8%-17.6%	0-10%	NA	NA	NA	31.3%	NA	NA
Obstruction >4-6 wk	11.2%	0-2.9%	NA	NA	6%-28%	NA	3%-7%	4%-8%
Obstruction requiring intervention	0-14.8%	0-2.1%	NA	0-2%	2%-10%	6.5%-18.8%	NA	NA

TVT, Gynecare TVT Retropubic System (Ethicon Women's Health and Urology, Somerville, NJ); TVT-O, Gynecare TVT Obturator System Tension-Free Support for Incontinence (Ethicon Women's Health and Urology); TVT-Secur, Gynecare TVT Secur System (Ethicon Women's Health and Urology); SPARC, SPARC Self-Fixating Sling System (American Medical Systems, Minnetonka, MN).
CIC, Clean intermittent catheterization; *NA,* not available.
From Nitti VW, ed. *Vaginal Surgery for the Urologist.* Philadelphia: Saunders; 2012.

development of irritative symptoms of frequency, urgency, and urge incontinence. Women may also present with a combination of voiding and storage symptoms. The clinical challenge is to determine whether these symptoms can be directly correlated to outlet obstruction secondary to either sling placement being too tight or overzealous tightening of suspension sutures.

Transient voiding dysfunction and retention can occur frequently and to a certain degree are expected to occur after certain types of anti-incontinence surgery. It is common for a patient to have retention for days to weeks after a biologic pubovaginal sling or certain suspension procedures. Patients with synthetic sling procedures done in isolation should void immediately postoperatively or shortly thereafter in most cases. Table 9-1 presents reported rates of obstruction after various sling and suspension procedures. When a surgical intervention for iatrogenic voiding dysfunction is believed to be necessary, controversy exists regarding the timing and techniques for these procedures. Preoperative cystourethroscopy should always be performed because the surgeon needs to ensure there is no sling material or sutures within the urethra or the bladder. Also, depending on the clinical situation, urodynamics studies may be helpful in documenting iatrogenic outlet obstruction as the cause for the patient's symptoms.

Traditionally, evaluation has been delayed for at least 3 months after surgery; this was based on literature following pubovaginal slings, colposuspension, or needle suspension where recurrent SUI after intervention was minimized by waiting at least 90 days. This waiting period that has been advocated for these traditional procedures has largely been abandoned for retropubic, transobturator, and single-incision synthetic midurethral sling procedures. Because of immobility of mesh and tremendous ingrowth of fibroblastic tissue by 2 weeks postoperatively, patients with retention or severe symptoms are unlikely to improve much beyond this time period. After retropubic and transobturator tape procedures, milder forms of temporary voiding dysfunction have been reported to resolve in 25% to 66% of patients in 1 to 2 weeks and 66% to 100% of patients by 6 weeks. Based on these data and our experience, waiting beyond 6 weeks for work-up and intervention seems unwarranted. Some authors would also argue that because 66% of patients should have symptoms resolve within 2 weeks, work-up and possible intervention are warranted at the 2-week mark or earlier after discussion with the patient about symptoms, level of bother, and willingness to risk possible intervention. In our practice, if a patient is unable to void spontaneously (i.e., urinary retention) within 1 week after a retropubic or transobturator tape procedure, we consider and discuss loosening the sling at that time, provided that a simultaneous pelvic organ prolapse repair was not done.

The work-up should include a focused history, physical examination, cystourethroscopy, and urodynamics testing in selected cases. Key points in the history are the patient's preoperative voiding status and the temporal relationship of new symptoms to the surgical procedure for SUI. Physical examination should focus on the angulation of the urethra. The urethra should be evaluated to determine if it appears to be hypersuspended and whether the urethral meatus appears to be pulled toward the pubic bone because a more vertical angle of the urethra suggests obstruction. However, most patients after synthetic midurethral sling procedures do not appear overcorrected. Patients should be examined for prolapse, urethral hypermobility, and recurrent SUI. As previously mentioned, cystourethroscopy should be performed to rule out any sling material in the urethra or bladder and to evaluate for any scarring, narrowing, occlusion, kinking, or deviation. It is also helpful to rule out any unsuspected pathology, such as a urethral diverticulum or bladder lesion.

Urodynamics testing can be performed if there is doubt regarding the diagnosis based on history, physical examination, and noninvasive testing (uroflow or post-void residual). There are no universally accepted urodynamics criteria for bladder outlet obstruction. Classic high pressure–low flow voiding dynamics confirm the diagnosis but are not always present even with significant obstruction owing to the differing voiding dynamics in women compared with men. For patients with complete retention shortly after surgery, urodynamics is of minimal diagnostic benefit. In a patient with retention, urodynamics can be used to identify detrusor instability and impaired compliance and confirm the diagnosis of obstruction. For a patient with predominately de novo storage symptoms with normal emptying, urodynamics can help identify or rule out obstruction. In these situations, many clinicians believe videourodynamics is preferable to standard urodynamics because the site of obstruction can be identified by fluoroscopy regardless of pressure and flow dynamics.

Case 1: Immediate Postoperative Retention after Retropubic Synthetic Midurethral Sling

A 37-year-old woman with fairly severe SUI undergoes a tension-free vaginal tape procedure that was uncomplicated. She is unable to void immediately after the procedure and is sent home with an indwelling Foley catheter. She comes to the office on postoperative day 3 for follow-up examination, and the catheter is removed and she is taught intermittent self-catheterization. At 1 week postoperatively, she is still not voiding spontaneously and performs self-catheterization every 3 to 5 hours with a yield of 300 to 500 mL. It is decided to attempt to loosen the sling in the operating room, with the goal being to maintain the continuity of the sling in the hope of maintaining continence. The procedure is performed under intravenous sedation and local infiltration of lidocaine. The patient is able to void spontaneously after the procedure and to date remains continent.

Discussion of Case

In women with postoperative urinary retention after retropubic and transobturator synthetic midurethral sling procedures, we advocate early intervention (within 7 to 14 days after surgery) because most patients should be able to void spontaneously within 72 hours. Early sling loosening allows one to perform a minimally invasive procedure under local anesthesia in the office setting or operating room. The goal is to stretch or loosen the sling maintaining the suburethral continuity of the sling material. Most likely cutting the sling during an early intervention such as this would result in a higher probability of recurrent stress incontinence. When the sling is firmly adherent to the posterior urethra, great care must be taken not to injure the urethra when loosening the sling.

Technique for Synthetic Sling Loosening in the Acute Setting (7 to 14 Days)

1. The patient is positioned in the lithotomy position, and the vagina is prepared in a sterile fashion.
2. The anterior vaginal wall is infiltrated with local anesthetic.
3. The surgeon cuts the suture used to close the vaginal wall and opens the prior incision.
4. The surgeon identifies the sling and hooks it with a right-angled clamp or other small clamp.
5. The surgeon spreads the clamp or applies downward traction to loosen the tape 1 to 2 cm.
6. The incision is closed with running absorbable suture (**Video 9-1**).

This technique is suitable to be performed in the office in a cooperative patient. However, it can be done in the operating room with very light intravenous sedation and local anesthesia in patients who are extremely anxious or intolerant of pain. It is best to perform this procedure before 14 days because after this time tissue ingrowth may prevent loosening, in which case it would most likely be preferable to cut the sling.

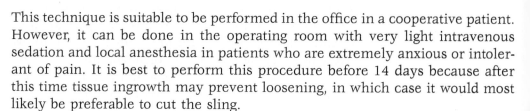

Case 2: Takedown of Retropubic Synthetic Sling at 4 Months Postoperatively

A 65-year-old woman presents approximately 4 months after vaginal hysterectomy with vaginal repairs of a cystocele and rectocele and a retropubic synthetic midurethral sling. She is still performing intermittent self-catheterization numerous times a day for significant voiding dysfunction. She voids 50 to 150 mL and persistently has residual volumes of 200 to 400 mL. The synthetic midurethral sling procedure was performed for suspected occult or potential SUI. Otherwise, she has no complications from the surgery and has had a very good result in regard to correction of prolapse. She denies any significant irritative symptoms in the form of frequency, urgency, or urge incontinence. The patient is becoming very frustrated with having to perform catheterization and desires resolution to the problem if available. Cystourethroscopy reveals no evidence of any injury to the urethra or bladder secondary from the previous surgery. Urodynamics studies note a stable detrusor to the volume of 450 mL with no evidence of any recurrent SUI. She is able to void only 120 mL during an attempted pressure flow study, but this is associated with significant abdominal straining and a detrusor contraction of 35 cm H_2O. After a detailed discussion of the potential surgical intervention, the patient agrees to a transvaginal excision of the suburethral portion of the synthetic mesh with the hope of having her voiding efficiency return to normal. She undergoes excision of the synthetic sling and has an immediate resumption of normal voiding with no evidence of recurrent SUI.

Discussion of Case

In this case, a synthetic sling was placed too tightly and resulted in voiding dysfunction. When managing occult incontinence, we prefer to use a transobturator or a single-incision sling because the literature seems to indicate there is a slightly higher risk for voiding dysfunction after a retropubic synthetic sling. However, this remains an area of controversy because more recent literature has noted that occult incontinence is more common in patients with pelvic organ prolapse than had previously been thought. The keys to success of takedown of a synthetic sling revolve around successfully identifying the sling and mobilizing it completely away from the entire urethra. We have seen numerous situations in which the sling is simply cut in the midline and the voiding dysfunction persists.

Steps for Takedown of a Synthetic Midurethral Sling

1. Repeat cystourethroscopy is performed in the operating room to ensure there is no evidence of sling penetration in the urethra or bladder.

2. Hydrodistention of the distal part of the anterior vaginal wall as previously described is performed.

3. A midline anterior vaginal wall incision is made with a scalpel, and the incision is taken down through the full thickness of the anterior vaginal wall. A gritty feeling detected with the knife indicates the location of the synthetic sling, appropriately identifying the location of the sling. If there is no gritty feeling detected with a knife, the tip of a finger can be used to palpate the area aggressively feeling for the synthetic polypropylene fibers. Frequently, the sling can be encased in scar tissue and can be under significant tension making it difficult to identify. A cystoscope or urethral sound can also be placed in the urethra with upward traction to help expose the exact location of the sling, isolating the axes of tension and indentation on the undersurface of the urethra.

4. After the sling is identified, we prefer to cut it in the midline with scissors and sharply lyse it away from the urethra all the way back to the inferior pubic ramus on each side. Another technique involves passing a right-angled clamp between the urethra and the sling, placing a clamp on each side of the exposed sling and cutting it in the midline, and then completing the lysis (Figures 9-1 and 9-2). If the sling is extremely tight, it can be isolated lateral to the urethra to avoid urethral injury. The mobilization of the sling off the

Figure 9-1 Technique for cutting synthetic midurethral sling. The sling is identified, and a right-angled clamp is placed between the sling and the urethra. The sling is cut in the midline.

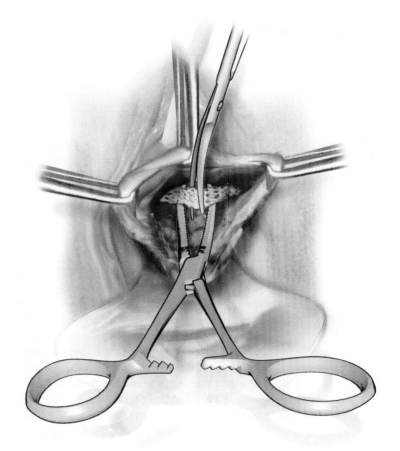

Figure 9-2 Technique for sharp dissection of sling off the posterior urethra. The synthetic sling sometimes is tightly adhered to the posterior urethra, and the surgeon is unable to pass a clamp safely between the sling and the urethra. The sling is cut in the midline, and sharp dissection is used to mobilize it off the urethra.

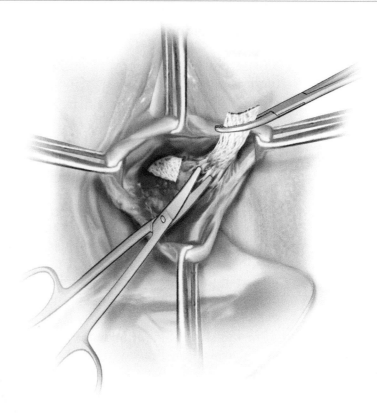

urethra is only to the level of the endopelvic fascia; this preserves lateral support of the urethra because the retropubic space is not entered, and it is hoped the likelihood of recurrent SUI is decreased (Figure 9-3; **Video 9-2**).

5. Surgeons should always obtain pathologic confirmation of the lysed portion of the synthetic sling because this documents a portion of the sling was cut in case the procedure was unsuccessful in completely resolving the voiding dysfunction.

6. The urethra should always be inspected very closely for any injury. In cases where the sling is deep to the periurethral fascia, it can be ingrown into the wall of the urethra, and excising the sling may result in an unexpected urethrotomy. In the event of this injury, the urethral defect should be closed in layers with a fine delayed-absorbable suture and the bladder continuously drained postoperatively for 7 to 10 days.

Case 3: Takedown of Synthetic Single-Incision Sling

A 45-year-old healthy woman with signs and symptoms of uncomplicated SUI elected to undergo placement of a single-incision minisling. Immediately after sling placement, the patient develops small volume urinary frequency, urgency, and urinary retention and failed her voiding trial after surgery. She is initiated on self-intermittent catheterization and followed for 2 weeks after surgery with no improvement in symptoms or dysfunctional voiding. On physical examination, the sling is not palpable, and the vaginal incision has healed without any sling exposure. Post-void residual measurement is 450 mL. After counseling the patient on possible options, including expectant management and observation, she elects to undergo an intraoperative lysis of her sling. During the procedure, the vaginal incision is recognized and opened along the previous suture line. The sling

Figure 9-3 A, Technique for takedown of a synthetic midurethral sling. The sling is identified, and a right-angled clamp is passed between the sling and the urethra. The edges of the sling are grasped with clamps, and the sling is cut at the midline. It is important to dissect the sling completely away from the urethra to ensure that the voiding dysfunction is resolved. **B,** The sling has been cut, and the edges of the sling remain on the vaginal side of the urogenital diaphragm.

(From Baggish MS, Karram MM, eds. Atlas of Pelvic Anatomy and Gynecology Surgery, *ed 3. St. Louis: Saunders; 2011.)*

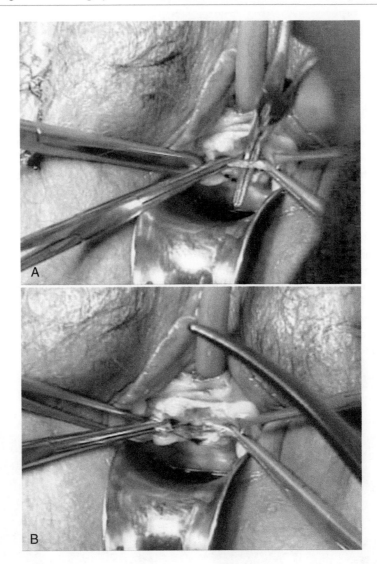

material is easily palpated and visualized in the submucosal tissue. It is correctly positioned in the midurethra but is visibly overtensioned. The sling is first engaged with a right-angled clamp by carefully sliding this between the sling and underlying urethra and then incised sharply with a scalpel. When incised, the sling noticeably springs apart and retracts into the periurethral tissues. The wound is closed with absorbable sutures. Postoperatively, she regains bladder function immediately and returns to baseline function, although she also has recurrence of SUI (**Video 9-3**).

Discussion of Case

In this case of bladder dysfunction resulting from an obstructing single-incision sling, sling lysis was performed with successful recovery of bladder function but also with recurrence of the initial SUI. This bladder dysfunction was certainly caused by overtensioning of the sling at the time of placement. Many clinicians would advocate for continued observation and expectant management, which may have been a reasonable option. Most episodes of voiding dysfunction resolve over several weeks with conservative management. Another proposed option for acute obstruction after midurethral sling placement is sling loosening, in which an attempt is made to pull down on the sling to "loosen" the degree of tensioning. Most single-incision sling devices have anchoring components to stabilize the material in situ. A loosening procedure is usually unsuccessful, necessitating formal sling lysis as in this case.

A 55-year-old woman presents with urinary retention and significant urge incontinence 3 months after an autologous rectus fascia pubovaginal sling. She is able to void only small amounts and needs to perform self-catheterization four times a day. Between catheterizations, she has episodes of urinary urge incontinence. Before surgery, she voided and emptied normally but had recurrent urinary tract infections. The rectus fascia pubovaginal sling was performed as a primary procedure because the patient refused a synthetic midurethral sling owing to concerns about the long-term placement of synthetic mesh. Postoperatively, her emptying has not improved since her catheter was removed approximately 10 weeks ago when she was instructed on self-catheterization. Cystoscopy is unremarkable: there is no evidence of any injury or foreign body within the bladder or the urethra. However, there is significant resistance to placement of the cystoscope at the level of the bladder neck consistent with an overzealous or tight pubovaginal sling. The patient consents to excision of the previously placed pubovaginal sling with the understanding that this may result in recurrence of SUI. The sling is successfully incised; however, the patient develops mild recurrent SUI over time.

Discussion of Case

In this case, the sling must be adjusted, cut, or taken down. The technique used to perform this procedure depends on the sling material and how it interacts with the patient's tissue. Certain autologous or allograft slings may aggressively incorporate with the surrounding tissue making it impossible to differentiate the sling material from the patient's tissue. In contrast, certain other biologic materials may be easily identifiable and easily dissected away from the patient's tissues and this is often unknown until the time of surgery. Whether or not the patient redevelops SUI or maintains continence is based on the degree of scarification, how aggressive the takedown is, and what sling material is used. Figure 9-4 demonstrates the technique of isolating and cutting a cadaveric fascia lata sling. There is significant release of tension around the urethra when the sling is cut in the midline.

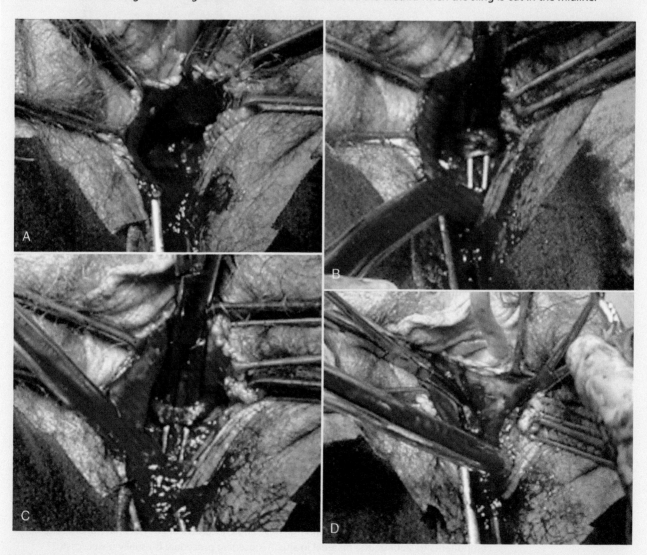

Figure 9-4 A, Cadaveric fascia lata sling causing urethral obstruction. **B,** A right-angled clamp has been passed between the sling and the urethra. **C,** Sling is being cut. **D,** Sling has been cut, and retracted ends are held in clamps.

(From Baggish MS, Karram MM, eds. Atlas of Pelvic Anatomy and Gynecology Surgery, *ed 3. St. Louis: Saunders; 2011.)*

Technique for Incision of a Biologic Bladder Neck Sling

1. Cystoscopy is performed intraoperatively to assess the urethra in the hope of identifying the exact area of obstruction and to rule out any previous injury to the urethra or the bladder.
2. An "inverted-U" or midline incision is made after injecting the anterior vaginal wall with a lidocaine/epinephrine solution.
3. Careful dissection to isolate the sling is performed. Injury to the urethra can be avoided by beginning dissection distally to identify normal urethra and then proceeding proximally to identify and isolate the sling keeping in mind that in most cases the sling is outside of the periurethral fascia.
4. The sling is isolated and should be separated off surrounding tissue sharply. Pubovaginal slings are usually wider than midurethral slings and usually require more dissection. The dissection can be facilitated by grasping the sling with a Kocher clamp on either side of the midline. If possible, a right-angled clamp is placed between the sling and the urethra, and the sling is cut in the midline (see Figure 9-4).
5. If no obvious biologic material is identified, one should proceed with an extensive vaginal urethrolysis as discussed later in this chapter with the goal being to create some urethral mobility above and beyond what was present before the surgery.
6. The vaginal incision is irrigated. Hemostasis is controlled as necessary, and the vaginal incision is closed with delayed absorbable sutures (**Video 9-4**).

Case 5: Retropubic and Vaginal Urethrolysis after Retropubic Suspension

A 75-year-old woman presents with a long-standing history of fairly severe urinary urgency, frequency, and urge incontinence. She also has had at least three documented urinary tract infections per year for the last several years. She has tried numerous antimuscarinic agents, which have failed to improve her overactive bladder symptoms. She had undergone a previous retropubic urethral suspension approximately 10 years before presentation. On pelvic examination, the urethra is noted to be markedly elevated and fixed with no bladder neck mobility. Post-void residual measurements are done on numerous occasions and are consistently between 200 and 300 mL. Cystourethroscopy notes a normal urethra and bladder. Videourodynamics testing is performed and notes obvious detrusor overactivity with voluntary voiding pressures of 42 cm H_2O with a maximum flow rate of 8 mL/s. There is an obvious area of obstruction caused by overelevation at the level of the proximal urethra. Based on the diagnosis of refractory detrusor overactivity in the face of outlet urethral obstruction and incomplete bladder emptying, urethrolysis is discussed and recommended. Both a vaginal and retropubic urethrolysis would be reasonable options. In this case, a better outcome most likely would occur from a retropubic takedown because the previous suspension was done retropubically. However, this is a controversial topic with the ultimate decision left to the discretion of the surgeon and his or her own clinical experience and expertise regarding urethrolysis. Both techniques for urethrolysis are discussed and demonstrated.

Technique for Retropubic or Abdominal Vesicourethrolysis

1. A large Foley catheter with a 30-mL balloon is placed inside the bladder.
2. A transverse, usually muscle-cutting incision (i.e., Cherney incision) is performed to facilitate exposure into the retropubic space (Figure 9-5).

Figure 9-5 Technique for Cherney muscle-cutting incision. **A,** A finger is taken around the entire belly of the rectus muscle. The finger should be behind the rectus muscle and in front of the peritoneum. The insertion of the muscle is taken off the back of the symphysis via electrocautery. **B,** The muscle has been completely detached from its insertion. **C,** Easy access to the retropubic space is apparent after both rectus muscles have been cut.

(From Baggish MS, Karram MM, eds. Atlas of Pelvic Anatomy and Gynecology Surgery, ed 3. St. Louis: Saunders; 2011.)

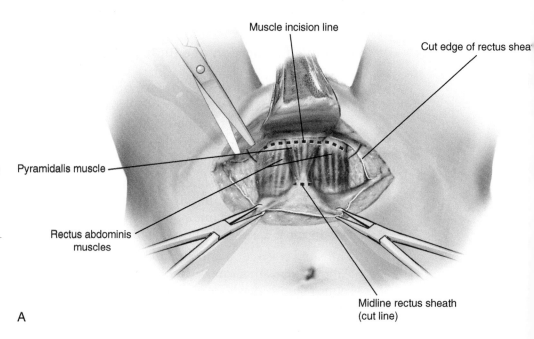

Muscle incision line

Cut edge of rectus sheath

Pyramidalis muscle

Rectus abdominis muscles

Midline rectus sheath (cut line)

A

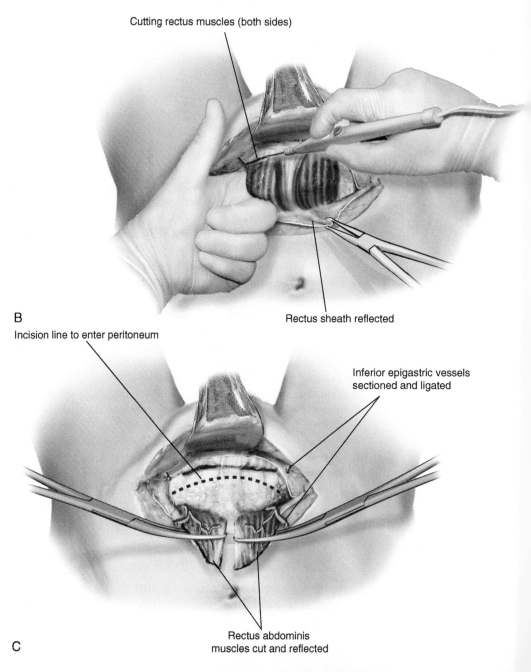

Cutting rectus muscles (both sides)

Rectus sheath reflected

B

Incision line to enter peritoneum

Inferior epigastric vessels sectioned and ligated

Rectus abdominis muscles cut and reflected

C

3. The bladder is taken down sharply off the back of the symphysis pubis all the way down the proximal urethra. It is best to make a high cystotomy to help in this dissection. It is important to mobilize the bladder and the proximal urethra completely from the back of the symphysis. The sutures or bone anchors from the previous suspension commonly are encountered and cut.

4. Dissection is extended laterally toward the pelvic sidewall and is taken down the level of the origin of the arcus tendineus fasciae pelvis or white line. This is also the lower margin of the obturator internus fascia (Figures 9-6 and 9-7).

5. When there is significant concern of rescarification of this area, it is sometimes beneficial to make a window in the peritoneum and bring a piece of omentum if available through the window to be placed between the back of the symphysis and the proximal urethra (Figure 9-8). Resuspension is almost never necessary. If a high cystocele is present in conjunction with the obstruction from the bladder neck suspension, a retropubic paravaginal

Figure 9-6 Retropubic vesicourethrolysis. A high extraperitoneal cystotomy has been made to facilitate sharp dissection of the bladder of the back of the symphysis pubis.

(From Baggish MS, Karram MM, eds. Atlas of Pelvic Anatomy and Gynecology Surgery, ed 3. St. Louis: Saunders; 2011.)

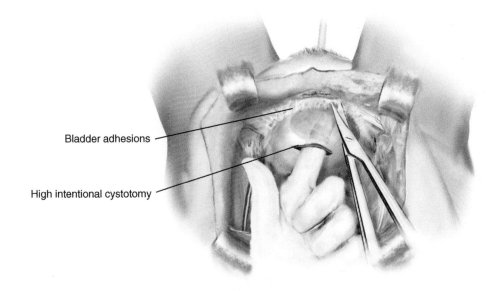

Bladder adhesions

High intentional cystotomy

Figure 9-7 Sharp dissection is continued down in the midline until the proximal one third of the urethra has been mobilized off the symphysis. Dissection is extended laterally down to the level of the paravaginal attachment at the arcus tendineus fasciae pelvis *(White line)*.

(From Baggish MS, Karram MM, eds. Atlas of Pelvic Anatomy and Gynecology Surgery, ed 3. St. Louis: Saunders; 2011.)

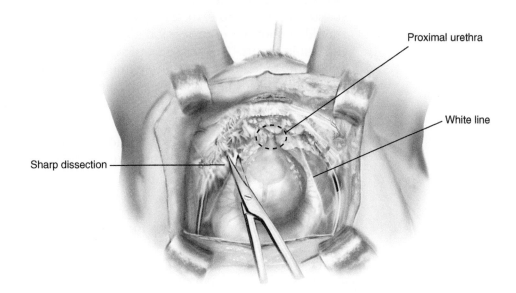

Proximal urethra

White line

Sharp dissection

Figure 9-8 To prevent rescarification in this area, a piece of omentum can be brought through a window in the peritoneum. The omentum is sutured at the midline to the lower aspect of the symphysis and laterally to the obturator fascia with numerous delayed-absorbable sutures.

(From Baggish MS, Karram MM, eds. Atlas of Pelvic Anatomy and Gynecology Surgery, *ed 3. St. Louis: Saunders; 2011.)*

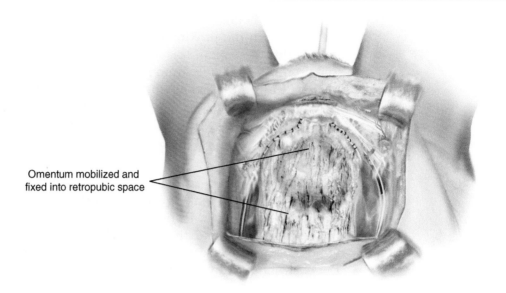

Omentum mobilized and fixed into retropubic space

defect repair can be performed simultaneously with the takedown (**Video 9-5**).

Technique for Vaginal Urethrolysis

1. A transurethral Foley catheter with a 30-mL balloon is placed within the bladder. Initial traction on the catheter with simultaneous vaginal palpation of bladder neck subjectively assesses the degree and extent of scarring elevation and fixation of the proximal urethra and bladder neck. The goal of vaginal urethrolysis is to create some mobility at the proximal urethra and bladder neck.

2. An "inverted-**U**" incision is made, and the vaginal wall is dissected off the underlying urethra and bladder neck (Figure 9-9). Allis clamps are used to grab the lateral part of the vaginal incision, and the dissections are extended laterally toward the inferior pubic ramus on each side.

3. Perforation of the urogenital diaphragm is performed using curved Mayo scissors pointing toward the ipsilateral shoulder. The tips of the scissors should penetrate the urogenital diaphragm at the inferior border of the inferior pubic ramus. The scissors are separated, and usually a finger is inserted and blunt takedown of all attachments of the urethra and bladder to the sidewall is performed bilaterally. Urethral mobility is subjectively assessed via traction on the Foley catheter. The dissection is continued until some urethral mobility has been created.

4. The entire area is irrigated, hemostasis is controlled, and the vaginal incision is closed usually with interrupted delayed-absorbable sutures (**Video 9-6**).

Postoperative Care After Sling Revision or Takedown

In most cases after sling loosening or incision, the patient is sent home without a catheter and is given perioperative antibiotics only. The patient should void

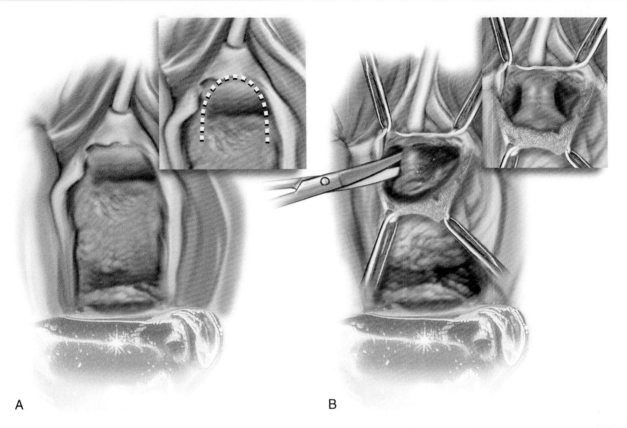

Figure 9-9 Technique of vaginal urethrolysis. **A,** "Inverted-U" incision is made on the vagina. **B,** Sharp dissection lateral to the bladder neck with sharp penetration of the urogenital diaphragm allows entry into the retropubic space with the possibility of creating some urethral mobility.

(From Baggish MS, Karram MM, eds. Atlas of Pelvic Anatomy and Gynecology Surgery, *ed 3. St. Louis: Saunders; 2011.)*

before leaving the office or recovery room. A catheter is left in situ in the event of urethral injury during sling incision or loosening or in cases of extensive urethrolysis. The length of catheterization depends on the size and nature of the injury and can range from 3 to 14 days. For patients who are hospitalized after transvaginal or retropubic urethrolysis, a vaginal packing and Foley catheter are left in overnight, and the catheter is left in place until vaginal packing is removed or until discharge if the patient is unable to void spontaneously while in the hospital. Ideally, the patient is instructed to perform clean intermittent catheterization, but if she is unwilling or unable, a Foley catheter is reinserted.

Outcomes

Very few objective data are available in the published literature regarding the results after sling loosening of synthetic midurethral slings. The few data available seem to indicate that such an intervention in these patients leads to resolution of their symptoms in 80% to 100% of cases. Resolution of voiding symptoms after sling incision has been reported to occur in 70% to 100% of cases, regardless of the type of sling. Resolution of voiding symptoms after transvaginal urethrolysis for all types of slings has been reported to be 33% to 92%. Time to intervention in all of these series was different, and this may play a role in the ultimate success of the intervention. Patient bother, morbidity of procedure, type of anti-incontinence procedure, and the patient's willingness to risk recurrent SUI should determine timing and treatment options.

SUI after sling loosening, sling incision, and transvaginal urethrolysis is a complication that should be discussed with all patients before intervention. The reported rates vary greatly, and the true rates are likely unknown owing to underreporting. Incidence of SUI after sling loosening, sling incision, or urethrolysis ranges from 0% to 39% with varying degrees of follow-up. We generally counsel patients by telling them they have a 15% to 30% chance of recurrence of SUI based on timing and type of takedown or sling revision.

Conclusion

Voiding dysfunction and/or retention occurs in the best of hands in a small percentage of patients after procedures to correct SUI. Ultimate timing and type of intervention for these problems should be individualized in the hope of meeting the patient's needs.

Suggested Readings

Barber MD, Gustilo-Ashby AM, Chen CC, Kaplan P, Paraiso MF, Walters MD. Perioperative complications and adverse events MONARC transobturator tape, compared with tension-free vaginal tape. *Am J Obstet Gynecol*. 2006;195:1820-1825.

Campeau L, Al-Afraa T, Corcos J. Evaluation and management of urinary retention after a suburethral sling procedure in women. *Curr Urol Rep*. 2008;9:412-418.

Chaikin DC, Rosenthal J, Blaivas JG. Pubovaginal fascial sling for all types of stress urinary incontinence: long-term analysis. *J Urol*. 1998;160:1312-1316.

Goldman HB. Simple sling incision for the treatment of iatrogenic urethral obstruction. *Urology*. 2003;62:714-718.

Karram MM, Segal JL, Vassallo BJ, Kleeman SD. Complications and untoward effects of the tension-free vaginal tape procedure. *Obstet Gynecol*. 2003;101:929-932.

Klutke C, Siegel S, Carlin B, Paszkiewicz E, Kirkemo A, Klutke J. Urinary retention after tension-free vaginal tape procedure: incidence and treatment. *Urology*. 2001;58:697-701.

Latthe PM, Fon R, Toozs-Hobson P. Transobturator and retropubic tape procedures in stress urinary incontinence: a systematic review and meta-analysis of effectiveness and complications. *BJOG*. 2007;114:522-531.

Leng WW, Davies BJ, Tarin T, et al. Delayed treatment of bladder outlet obstruction after sling surgery: association with irreversible bladder dysfunction. *J Urol*. 2004;172:1379-1381.

Lim JL, Cornish A, Carey MP. Clinical and quality of life outcomes in women treated by TVT-O procedure. *BJOG*. 2006;113:1315-1320.

Meschia M, Barbacini P, Ambrogi V, Pifarotti P, Ricci L, Spreafico L. TVT-Secur: a minimally invasive procedure for the treatment of primary stress urinary incontinence: one year data from a multicentre prospective trial. *Int Urogynecol J*. 2009;20:313-317.

Minassian V, Al-Badr A, Drutz HP, Lovatsis D. Tension-free vaginal tape, burch, and slings: are there predictors for early postoperative voiding dysfunction. *Int Urogynecol J*. 2004;15:183-187.

Mishra VC, Mishra N, Karim OMA, Motiwala HG. Voiding dysfunction after tension-free vaginal tape: a conservative approach is often successful. *Int Urogynecol J*. 2005;16:210-214.

Mitsui T, Tanaka H, Moriya K, Kakizaki H, Nonomura K. Clinical and urodynamic outcomes of pubovaginal sling procedure with autologous fascia for stress urinary incontinence. *Int J Urol*. 2007; 14:1076-1079.

Morgan TO Jr, Westney OL, McGuire EJ. Pubovaginal sling: 4-year outcome analysis and quality of life assessment. *J Urol*. 2000;163:1845-1848.

Niemczyk P, Klutke JJ, Carlin BI, Klutke CG. United States experience with tension-free vaginal tape procedure for urinary stress incontinence: assessment of safety and tolerability. *Tech Urol*. 2001;7: 261-265.

Nitti VW, Raz S. Obstruction following anti-incontinence procedures: diagnosis and treatment with transvaginal urethrolysis. *J Urol*. 1994;152:93-98.

Novi JM, Mulvihill BHK. Surgical intervention for stress urinary incontinence: comparison of midurethral sling procedures. *J Am Osteopath Assoc*. 2008;108:634-638.

Petrou SP, Brown JA, Blaivas JG. Suprameatal transvaginal urethrolysis. *J Urol.* 1999;161:1268-1271.

Rapp DE, Kobashi KC. The evolution of midurethral slings. *Nat Clin Pract Urol.* 2008;5:194-201.

Rardin CR, Rosenblatt PL, Kohli N, Miklos JR, Heit M, Lucente VR. Release of tension-free vaginal tape for the treatment of refractory postoperative voiding dysfunction. *Obstet Gynecol.* 2002;100: 898-902.

Rosenblum N, Nitti VW. Posturethral suspension obstruction. *Curr Opin Urol.* 2001;11:411-416.

Segal J, Steele A, Vassallo B, et al. Various surgical approaches to treat voiding dysfunction following anti-incontinence surgery. *Int Urogynecol J.* 2006;17:372-377.

Sokol AI, Jelovsek JE, Walters MD, Paraiso MFR, Barber MD. Incidence and predictors of prolonged urinary retention after TVT with and without concurrent prolapse surgery. *Am J Obstet Gynecol.* 2005;192:1537-1543.

South MM, Wu JM, Webster GD, Weidner AC, Roelands JJ, Amundsen CL. Early v late midline sling lysis results in greater improvement in lower urinary tract symptoms. *Am J Obstet Gynecol.* 2009;200:564.e1-564.e5.

Starkman JS, Duffy JW 3rd, Wolter CE, Kaufman MR, Scarpero HM, Dmochowski RR. The evolution of obstruction-induced overactive bladder symptoms following urethrolysis for female bladder outlet obstruction. *J Urol.* 2008;179:1018-1023.

Tamussino K, Hanzal E, Kolle D, Ralph G, Riss P. The Austrian tension-free vaginal tape registry. *Int Urogynecol J.* 2001;12(Suppl 2):S28-S29.

Walid MS, Heaton RL. A minimally invasive technique for relaxing overtensioned midurethral slings. *Arch Gynecol Obstet.* 2009;280(4):691-692.

Wheeler II TL, Richter HE, Greer WJ, et al. Predictors of success with postoperative voiding trials after a midurethral sling procedure. *J Urol.* 2008;179:600-604.

Bulk-Enhancing Agents for Stress Incontinence: Indications and Techniques

10

Roger Dmochowski, M.D.
W. Stuart Reynolds, M.D.
Melissa R. Kaufman, M.D.

 Video

10-1 Cystoscopic Injection of Urethral
Bulking Agent (Coaptite)

Introduction

In the intervening 70 years since its first description, various materials have been used as agents in urethral injection therapy (UIT) for the treatment of urinary incontinence. The peak interest in UIT occurred in the mid-1990s to the early 2000s; presumably because of mediocre clinical results, especially long term, and the increase in popularity of alternative treatment options, the initial enthusiasm has waned. However, UIT still has a role in treatment of stress urinary incontinence (SUI) because it is minimally invasive, well tolerated, and beneficial, especially in the short-term. It can be easily administered in the outpatient setting with very little associated morbidity. Appropriate patient selection is paramount because in the right patient, urethral injection bulking therapy can play an important role in treating SUI.

History

UIT for urinary incontinence was first reported in the 1930s and included materials such as sodium morrhuate, paraffin wax, and other sclerosing agents. The technique gained greater widespread acceptance with the use of polytetrafluoroethylene (Teflon) in the 1970s and 1980s along with concomitant development of the concept of intrinsic sphincter deficiency (ISD), a characterization of SUI without urethral hypermobility. Additional agents that emerged at that time included autologous fat and collagen. Eventually polytetrafluoroethylene and fat were abandoned because of safety concerns; however, collagen would become and remained until recently the gold standard agent for injection therapy. In the last 2 decades, numerous synthetic and biologic agents have entered the market, some with encouraging results and others with significant safety issues (e.g., Tegress™). Finally, with the advent of efficacious, minimally invasive midurethral slings (see Chapters 6-8), popularity and perceived need for UIT for ISD have waned.

Patient Selection

Traditionally, UIT has been reserved for patients specifically with isolated ISD (i.e., urodynamically proven low abdominal leakpoint pressure [<100 cm H_2O], limited urethral mobility, and absence of detrusor instability). With greater experience using UIT, a broader range of patients with SUI have been treated, and the technology can be applied to all types of SUI.

Good candidates for UIT generally include patients who:

1. Are poor surgical candidates
2. Are elderly and at greatest risk of retention after a sling procedure
3. Must continue anticoagulation therapy at all times
4. Desire nonsurgical therapy using only local anesthesia
5. Are unable to follow postoperative activity limitations required after anti-incontinence procedures
6. Desire more children in the future
7. Have SUI and poor bladder emptying
8. Have had suboptimal symptom improvement after sling surgery (i.e., possible salvage procedure)

An important role for UIT may be as an adjuvant treatment option after an incomplete response to more definitive treatment. Durable responses are possible in patients with persistent SUI after a failed incontinence procedure or pelvic organ prolapse surgery who were treated with collagen injection. Additionally, UIT may be considered as a "first-line" therapy, with more definitive intervention reserved (e.g., midurethral sling) for patients who fail UIT. Efficacy of subsequent incontinence procedures does not seem to be affected by previous UIT.

Finally, managing patient expectations is very important. Most women have expectations that their urine leakage will be eliminated by a single anti-incontinence surgical procedure. However, patients need to understand that UIT should be viewed as a process, rather than a single intervention, and multiple injections may be required to achieve satisfactory results.

Injection Agents—"Ideal Agent"

The success of a particular agent for UIT depends on the composition of the material, the usability of the material (ease of preparation and implantation), and the host environment where it is implanted (optimized hormonal environment, integrity of urethral mural components, and intact periurethral fascia). The ideal bulking agent should be nonimmunogenic, permanent, nonmigratory, nonerosive, and noninflammatory; be easily stored, handled, and injected; be painless; have no long-term side effects; and possess a high safety profile. Because no existing agent satisfies all these requirements, the search continues for improved materials and delivery methods.

Table 10–1 Urethral bulking agents

Brand Name	Manufacturer	Material Composition
Contigen	CR Bard, Covington, GA	Bovine collagen
Macroplastique	Uroplasty Inc, Minneapolis, MN	Silicone hydrogel
Durasphere	Boston Scientific, Natick, MA	Carbon beads
Coaptite	Boston Scientific	Calcium hydroxyapatite
Deflux, Zuidex	Q-Med, Uppsala, Sweden	Dextronomer/hyaluronic acid copolymer
Bulkamid, Aquamid	Contura International, Soeborg, Denmark	Polyacrylamide hydrogel

Several agents have been developed and tested for UIT. Three commercially available bulking agents are available at the present time (Table 10-1). Bovine collagen has historically been the benchmark agent in that the U.S. Food and Drug Administration requires efficacy studies comparing new agents with collagen for consideration of approval. Additional materials used as bulking agents are composed of various biologic and synthetic materials, including carbon, silicone, calcium hydroxyapatite, and copolymers of hyaluronic acid and polyacrylamide.

Particle migration is a safety as well as efficacy concern, and small size (generally <100 μ) and high-pressure injection systems increase the likelihood of material migration and embolus. These practical considerations have led to many material and delivery device modifications to accommodate larger size particles and lower pressure injection systems.

Injection Technique

Several injection techniques have been described for UIT, but the most common are transurethral and periurethral approaches. Retropubic, antegrade techniques have been described for male urethral injection but are not commonly performed. Instruments and injection devices are both universal and proprietary, depending on the material used. Most materials are delivered in either preloaded syringes for use with generic rigid cystourethroscope injection needles or preloaded needle injection devices for use with generic rigid scope sets.

The transurethral technique involves injection of the bulking material submucosally via a needle inserted through a conventional cystourethroscope under direct visual guidance. The periurethral injection technique involves injecting material periurethrally with a needle or specialty injector device placed percutaneously from a perimeatal injection site. The needle is positioned submucosally under direct endoscopic vision in the urethra. The target of implantation via either technique is placement of the material in the urethral wall distal to the bladder neck in the midurethra to proximal urethra (Figure 10-1).

Most patients can be injected under local anesthesia, with topical lidocaine jelly in the urethra, direct submucosal lidocaine injection, or periurethral infiltration with injectable lidocaine. The patient is placed in the dorsal lithotomy position and prepared in a typical sterile fashion as for a cystoscopic procedure. Antibiotic prophylaxis can be considered as with any office-based cystoscopic procedure.

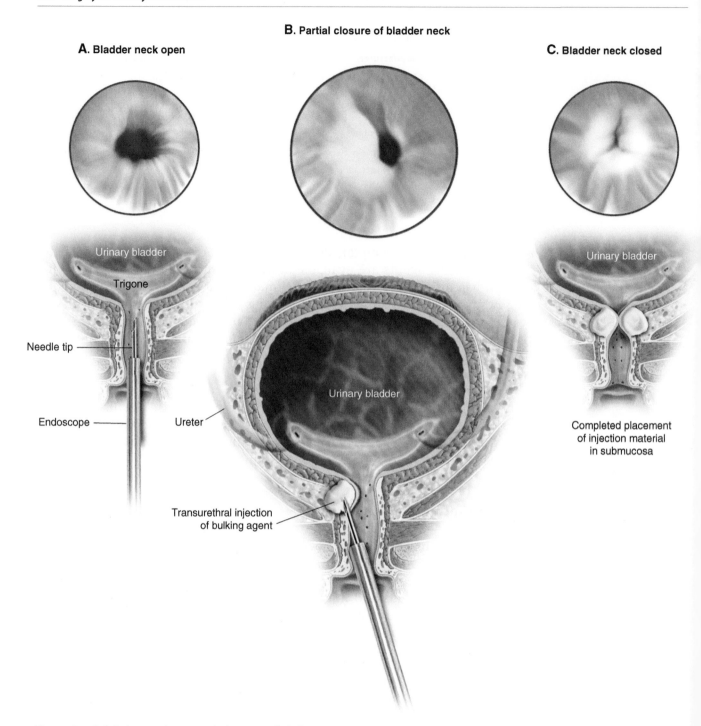

B. Partial closure of bladder neck

A. Bladder neck open

C. Bladder neck closed

Urinary bladder

Trigone

Urinary bladder

Needle tip

Urinary bladder

Endoscope

Ureter

Completed placement
of injection material
in submucosa

Transurethral injection
of bulking agent

Figure 10-1 A-C, Techniques for transurethral injection of a bulking agent.

Case Scenario

A 73-year-old woman presents with a several-year history of mild to moderate urinary incontinence associated with activity for which she has to wear two to three sanitary pads per day. She had undergone a "bladder tack" or suspension 25 years ago but has had no other pelvic or vaginal surgery. She voids with a good stream and empties to completion with a post-void residual of 50 mL. On examination, she has a well-supported anterior vaginal wall with minimal mobility of the urethra, and the sign of SUI is easily demonstrated with coughing in the supine position. She is otherwise well except for hypertension and hypercholesterolemia and is physically active. After discussion of all options, she is not interested in invasive surgical treatment but is interested in undergoing urethral bulking treatment.

Transurethral Injection Technique

1. *Analgesia.* Urethral bulking agents are typically injected under local analgesia administered at the time of treatment, either in a topical or an injectable form. Immediately before bulking agent injection, 1% lidocaine or 25% bupivacaine can be injected transurethrally, or a periurethral block can be administered.

2. *Cystoscopy.* The cystoscope and injection needle are inserted into the urethra under direct vision to the level of the bladder neck. The cystoscope is slightly withdrawn to the midurethra so that the needle can be inserted within the submucosa tissue layer to implant the material at the bladder neck and proximal urethra. A 0-, 12-, or 30-degree lens should be used.

3. *Injection of local analgesic.* If injectable lidocaine is to be used, it is injected first. This helps not only with analgesia but also with hydrodistention of the periurethral tissues and submucosa to allow easier agent injection.

4. *Injection of material.* Injection of bulking agents generally proceeds with several injection sites within the same level of the urethra and bladder neck (e.g., 3-o'clock, 9-o'clock, 12-o'clock, 4-o'clock, and 8-o'clock positions) and with sufficient material so that horizontal or concentric coaptation of the urethral mucosa is achieved with material injection. Injection must be slow enough so that the tissue can accommodate the material without extrusion of the material either from a new rent in the mucosa or from the needle puncture site after the needle is withdrawn (**Video 10-1** ; see Figure 10-1).

Periurethral Injection Technique

1. *Analgesia.* A perimeatal block of injectable lidocaine is performed initially.

2. *Cystoscopy.* Cystourethroscopy is performed initially to help with localization of the injection needle for accurate deposition of the material at the bladder neck and proximal urethra.

3. *Needle insertion and localization.* Bulking agent material is generally injected at two circumferential positions at the bladder neck and proximal urethra, at the 4-o'clock and 8-o'clock positions. The injection needle or device is inserted just lateral to the urethral meatus and advanced within the wall of the urethra through the lamina propria to the proximal urethra and bladder neck area. Gentle rocking of the injection needle can help to localize the needle tip and confirm the proper location of injection site. Submucosal instillation of methylene blue has also been used to assist in needle localization. A 15-degree angled injection needle (so-called bent-needle technique) can also facilitate needle localization and ease of injection. Care must be taken to avoid any puncture of the mucosa, or extrusion of the injected material can occur.

4. *Material injection.* The bulking agent is injected slowly and smoothly to allow tissue accommodation of the material, with the development of raised mounds of mucosa until apposition is achieved. If extrusion of material develops, the needle can be repositioned more anteriorly, and injection can be resumed. After injection of one side is performed, the needle is removed and reinserted on the contralateral side. Enough material is injected so that coaptation is achieved.

Outcomes and Complications

Outcomes treating SUI with UIT have historically been modest, particularly long-term (i.e., >12 months) outcomes. Generally, approximately 25% to 33% of patients are dry or cured, 33% to 50% are improved, and 25% to 33% have no improvement. After approximately 1 year, the success rates decrease dramatically for most materials, but some studies have shown continued efficacy for 2 years. Retreatment or reinjection may be necessary for patients who initially respond but have recurrence of symptoms.

Complications are rare. Acute urinary retention is a particularly difficult scenario immediately after UIT. Generally, urinary retention occurs in 15% of patients and is universally temporary, lasting 1 to 3 days. There is theoretical concern over indwelling urethral catheters causing molding of the injected agent within the wall of the urethra, compromising the desired benefit of the UIT. Intermittent self-catheterization with a small-caliber catheter is generally recommended as the treatment of urinary retention in this setting. Retention is most commonly seen after injection of relatively large quantities of material, particularly when injected with circumferential coaptation. To avoid this complication, some clinicians have advocated a staged injection procedure, whereby material is injected in one location at one setting, and the remaining circumferential locations are injected at procedures spaced 1 month apart. For a treatment requiring three injections (e.g., 3-o'clock, 6-o'clock, and 9-o'clock), this equates to three procedures spread over 3 months. Full efficacy is delayed, but the risk of urinary retention is diminished.

Other complications are uncommon or minor in severity. Transient de novo urgency and frequency can develop in 5% of patients. Hematuria and dysuria are common symptoms immediately after injection. Urinary tract infections can occur after injection. Some instances of bulking material erosion into the urethra, bladder, or vagina have been described, as have the formation of sterile abscesses at the sight of injection.

Tips and Tricks

1. Optimize visualization of the urethra before injection.
2. Inject as rapidly as feasible without compromising material placement.
3. Use the same needle puncture site for anesthesia and material placement so that the local anesthetic distends the urethral submucosa before material injection.
4. Never overinject; usually 1.5 to 3 mL per injection session is sufficient.

Troubleshooting

1. If material extrusion occurs during injection, remove the injection needle and reinsert it at another site.
2. If retention occurs after injection and the patient is unable to perform clean intermittent self-catheterization, use a 10F or 12F catheter for continuous drainage for a short time.

Suggested Readings

Chapple CR, Wein AJ, Brubaker L, et al. Stress incontinence injection therapy: what is best for our patients? *Eur Urol.* 2005;48:552-565.

Keegan PE, Atiemo K, Cody J, McClinton S, Pickard R. Periurethral injection therapy for urinary incontinence in women. *Cochrane Database Syst Rev.* 2007;(3):CD003881.

Kotb AF, Campeau L, Corcos J. Urethral bulking agents: techniques and outcomes. *Curr Urol Rep.* 2009;10:396-400.

Starkman JS, Scarpero H, Dmochowski RR. Emerging periurethral bulking agents for female stress urinary incontinence: is new necessarily better? *Curr Urol Rep.* 2006;7:405-413.

Sacral Neuromodulation

W. Stuart Reynolds, M.D.
Melissa R. Kaufman, M.D.
Roger Dmochowski, M.D.

 Videos

11-1 Percutaneous Nerve Evaluation   **11-3** Stage II Implant
11-2 Stage I Implant

Introduction

Sacral neuromodulation (SNM) received approval from the U.S. Food and Drug Administration in 1997 (InterStim; Medtronic, Inc, Minneapolis, MN). SNM is indicated for the treatment of refractory urge urinary incontinence, frequency-urgency syndrome, and idiopathic urinary retention and chronic fecal incontinence. Although the exact mechanism of action has not been fully determined, SNM appears to modulate bladder behavior through electrical stimulation of somatic afferent axons in the spinal roots, which modulate voiding and continence reflex pathways in the central nervous system, likely by inhibiting interneuronal transmission in the bladder reflex pathway (Amend et al., 2011a). Neuromodulation also may have a direct effect on the pelvic floor.

The InterStim device has three components: a battery-powered neurostimulator (also known as the implantable pulse generator [IPG]), an extension cable, and a tined electrical lead (Figure 11-1). The tined lead is a semipermanent, insulated electrical stimulation lead with four contact points near the tip (quadripolar) and four plastic collapsible projections (tines), which help to anchor the lead to the surrounding tissue. The IPG is a remotely programmable, battery-operated device that generates an electrical stimulus transferred to the lead contact points. With SNM, the electrical lead is implanted in close proximity to the third sacral nerve root (S3) at the level of the S3 spinal foramen (Figure 11-2). Stimulation of the S3 nerve root has demonstrated the best efficacy for SNM because S3 provides innervation to the bladder itself. Appropriate positioning of the electrical lead is verified by motor or sensory responses to electrical stimulation at the time of implantation (Figure 11-3). The S3 nerve root and neighboring S2 and S4 roots exhibit characteristic responses to electrical stimulation (Table 11-1). Ipsilateral great toe plantar flexion and pelvic floor "bellows" response are the predictable motor responses seen with S3 stimulation.

Most commonly, the device is implanted after a test phase (i.e., nerve evaluation) initially confirms therapeutic response. The test phase may be accomplished using a temporary, disposable lead implanted in the office as part of a basic evaluation (i.e., percutaneous or peripheral nerve evaluation [PNE]) or with a tined lead as part of a planned two-phase procedure. For PNE, a

Figure 11-1 InterStim device composed of a battery-powered, remote-programmable neurostimulator (IPG), a semipermanent tined electrical lead, and an insulated extension cable.

(Courtesy Medtronic, Inc, Minneapolis, MN.)

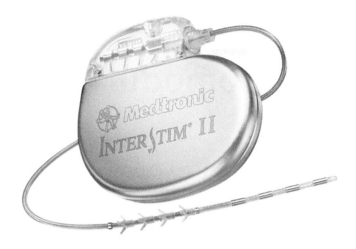

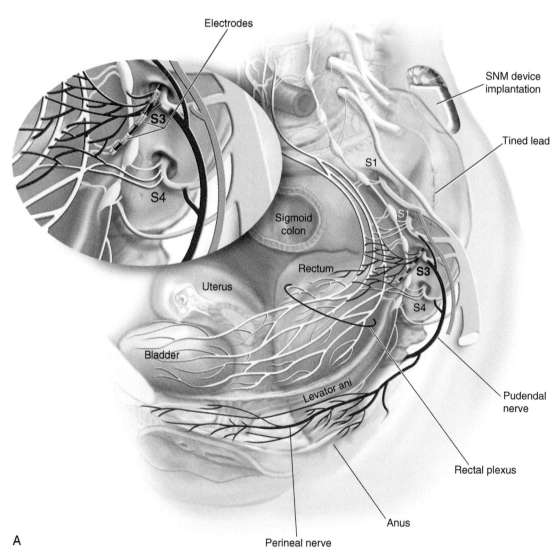

A

Figure 11-2 Final position of the four electrical contact points of the stimulation lead in close proximity to the third sacral nerve root (S3) and the four plastic projections or tines embedded in and securing the lead to the tissue overlying the sacral foramen. **A,** Lateral view.

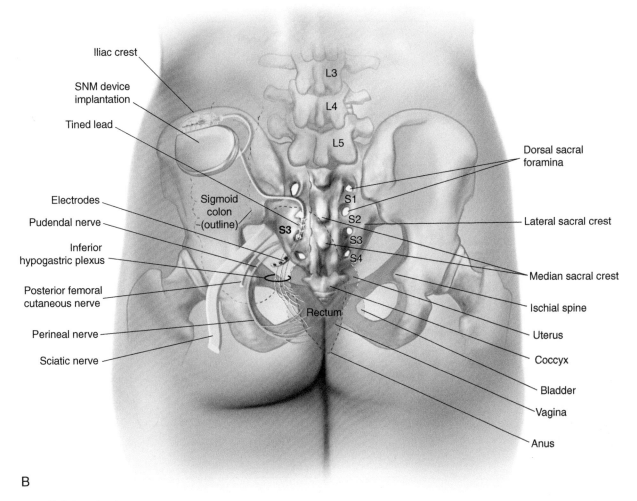

Iliac crest
SNM device implantation
Tined lead
Electrodes
Pudendal nerve
Inferior hypogastric plexus
Posterior femoral cutaneous nerve
Perineal nerve
Sciatic nerve

Sigmoid colon (outline)
S3
Rectum

L3
L4
L5
S1
S2
S3
S4

Dorsal sacral foramina
Lateral sacral crest
Median sacral crest
Ischial spine
Uterus
Coccyx
Bladder
Vagina
Anus

B

Figure 11-2, cont'd B, Posterior view.

Table 11–1 Sacral nerve root responses to electrical stimulation			
Nerve Root	**Pelvic Floor**	**Ipsilateral Lower Extremity**	**Sensation**
S2	Anal sphincter contraction	Lateral leg rotation, plantar flexion of entire foot	Sensations in leg or buttock
S3	"Bellows" response of pelvic floor (levator muscles contraction)	Great toe flexion	"Pulling" in rectum, scrotum, or vagina
S4	"Bellows" response of pelvic floor	None	"Pulling" in rectum only

temporary, unipolar electrical lead is percutaneously implanted under local analgesia, typically in the office setting, and a short-term trial period (7 days) ensues to confirm response. With positive results, the temporary lead is easily removed, and the patient can progress directly to single-stage InterStim implantation (i.e., quadripolar lead and IPG) in the operating room. If results are inconclusive, an advanced evaluation approach may be tried using implantation of a tined, quadripolar lead (discussed later).

Alternatively, the InterStim system may be implanted in first-time patients with a staged, two-step process involving an initial percutaneous placement of the tined lead with an external impulse generator for a short trial period

Figure 11-3 Different responses to stimulation of S2 to S4.

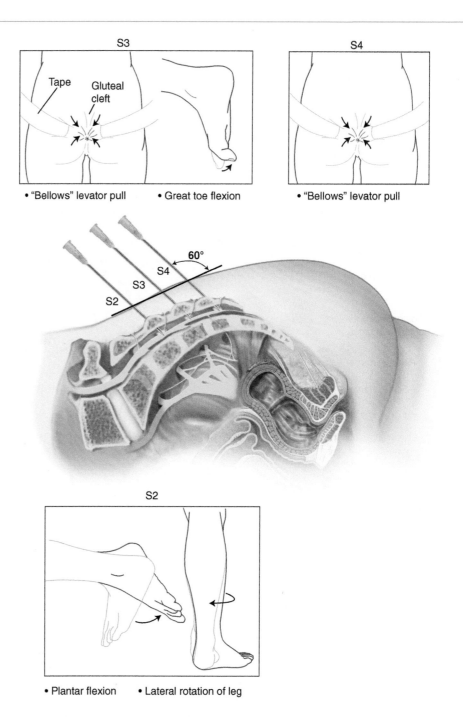

S3

Tape   Gluteal cleft

• "Bellows" levator pull   • Great toe flexion

S4

• "Bellows" levator pull

60°

S4
S3
S2

S2

• Plantar flexion   • Lateral rotation of leg

followed by permanent implantation of the IPG device in patients who respond to the trial period. The tined electrical lead placement is typically done with fluoroscopic guidance but may also be done without, using palpable bony landmarks. A temporary, external electrical stimulator is attached, and a clinical trial period of 1 to 4 weeks ensues, during which the patient evaluates his or her response to the therapy. If appropriate benefit occurs (defined as a >50% improvement in symptoms as measured by a voiding diary), the IPG is connected to the previously placed lead and surgically implanted in the upper buttocks during a second surgical stage procedure. If there is not a significant response, the implanted lead is removed without implanting an IPG. Adjustments to the impulse generator settings can be made with a remote programming device.

Case Scenario

 (Video 11-1)

A 55-year-old woman who has had urge incontinence for more than 3 years, without known neurologic disease or other significant morbidities, with a normal physical examination, and with negative urinalysis and cytology requests therapy for her symptoms. She has received two different antimuscarinic agents, each for 1 month, with dose escalation being used and with no significant reduction in symptoms despite medication combination with optimized behavioral therapy. Urodynamics reveals a bladder capacity of 175 mL, with detrusor overactivity occurring at 100 mL with incontinence and no evidence of obstructed voiding and minimal post-void residual. Diagnostic cystoscopy is unremarkable. The patient is very bothered by her symptoms and desires an attempt at more definitive therapy if possible. After a detailed discussion of options, including botulinum toxin (Botox) injection and SNM, she decides to proceed with a PNE test stimulation.

Sacral Neuromodulation Implantation Technique

Percutaneous or Peripheral Nerve Evaluation

1. *Patient positioning, setup, and analgesia.* Temporary lead placement during PNE may be performed in the outpatient clinic under local analgesia. The patient is positioned prone on the procedure table with slight flexion at the hips. The patient's shoes and socks are also removed to allow observation of the feet. The nonsterile ground pad is affixed to the skin away from the site of lead placement (sterile field). The skin overlying the sacrum, buttocks, and perineum is sterilely cleansed, and surgical drapes are placed to allow visualization and inspection of the buttocks and gluteal crease. Analgesia is achieved through infiltration of the skin and subcutaneous tissues down to the bone in the vicinity of the desired sacral foramina with local anesthetic (e.g., lidocaine or bupivacaine).

2. *S3 localization and lead placement.* To locate the S3 foramen, anatomic landmarks or fluoroscopy may be used (Figure 11-4). When the approximate location of the S3 foramen is identified, a foramen needle is inserted percutaneously into the foramen at a 60-degree angle relative to the skin. The test stimulator is connected to the foramen needle via the test stimulation cable, and stimulation is applied. With electrical stimulation applied, the clinician observes for responses to stimulation (see Table 11-1 and Figure 11-3). If the desired responses are not seen, the needle may be moved up and down to change the depth, or a foramen needle may be placed on the contralateral side. If responses are consistent with different sacral nerves (i.e., S2 or S4), the needle may be reinserted into the appropriate foramen and retested. If the desired responses are seen, the test stimulation lead is inserted into the foramen needle until the lead electrode exits the needle tip (determined by markings on the lead). The lead is retested for appropriate responses, and if confirmed, the foramen needle is removed over the lead, leaving the lead in place in the S3 foramen.

3. *Completion.* After the lead is deployed, the test stimulation cable is attached to the test lead and affixed to the skin using a transparent dressing. The test stimulator is set up for patient home use by attaching the test cable to the stimulator and affixing the grounding pad, securing both to the patient with adhesive tape.

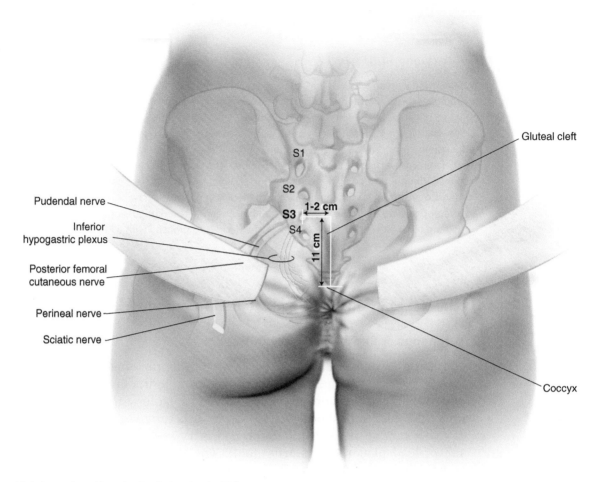

Figure 11-4 Anatomic and bony landmarks locating the S3 foramen.

4. *Lead removal.* After the evaluative interval, the lead is removed by removing the adhesive dressings and withdrawing the lead from the skin incision with gentle traction.

Almost any patient may be screened for SNM with a PNE trial or stage 1 lead implantation, although lead implantation generally is more successful than PNE. If a patient fails PNE, surgical lead implantation may be attempted as a salvage procedure. If not, other treatment modalities should be considered. In patients in whom sacral spinal anatomy may be distorted (e.g., malformations, trauma, or surgery), placement of a tined, quadripolar lead during an advanced, staged evaluation under fluoroscopic guidance may be more beneficial than PNE testing.

When PNE followed by stage I implantation was studied in a group of 69 patients with overactive bladder, 48% had a positive response to PNE, and 73% had a positive response to stage I implantation, suggesting that an additional 25% of patients may be salvaged with stage I implantation (Leong et al., 2011a). Using administrative health care claims for patients undergoing PNE or stage I testing, Cameron et al. (2011) documented that only 45.8% of Medicare patients and 24.1% of privately insured patients underwent IPG placement after a PNE trial (vs. 35.4% of Medicare and 50.9% of privately insured patients after stage I lead placement).

Electrical Lead Placement, First Stage

 (Video 11-2)

1. *Anesthesia.* SNM devices may be implanted with general or local anesthesia with sedation. Pharmacologic paralysis should be avoided because testing for motor nerve response is critical to verifying correct positioning of the electrical lead. Some practitioners advocate insertion in the nonsedated state so that the patient can report sensory cues during implantation.

2. *Patient positioning and setup.* The patient is placed prone, ensuring that adequate padding for pressure points is provided. Rolled towels or foam is used to support the abdomen and chest, and the shoulders must rest in a neutral position. A wide surgical area is sterilely cleansed from the midback to the upper thighs and laterally to the midaxillary line (Figure 11-5). Surgical drapes are placed to allow visualization and inspection of the buttocks and gluteal crease; the use of a clear, plastic drape can facilitate this. In addition, the feet and ankles are left undraped (Figure 11-6).

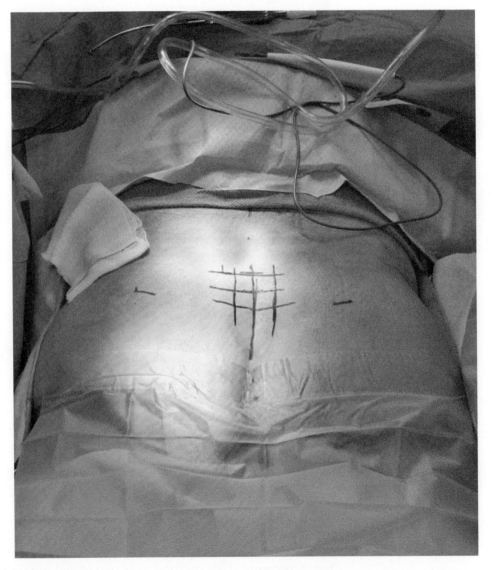

Figure 11-5 A wide surgical area is sterilely cleansed from the midback to the upper thighs and laterally to the midaxillary line, and surgical drapes are placed to allow visualization and inspection of the buttocks and gluteal crease; the use of a clear, plastic drape can facilitate this.

Figure 11-6 The patient's feet and ankles are left undraped to allow for observation for motor responses.

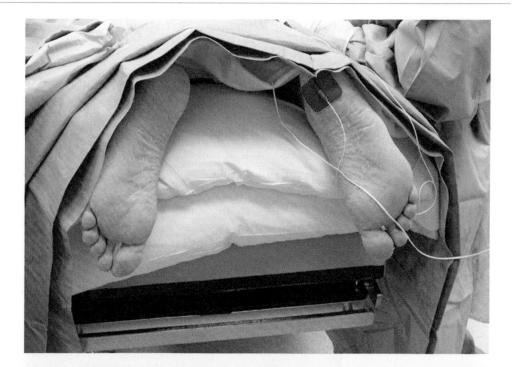

Figure 11-7 Fluoroscopic image of crosshair method for sacral foramen localization. The vertical needle is placed over the midline of the patient's spine. The horizontal needle is placed on a line formed by the ischial spines. The S3 foramen is one fingerbreadth (1.5 to 2 cm) away from the cross junction of the needles.

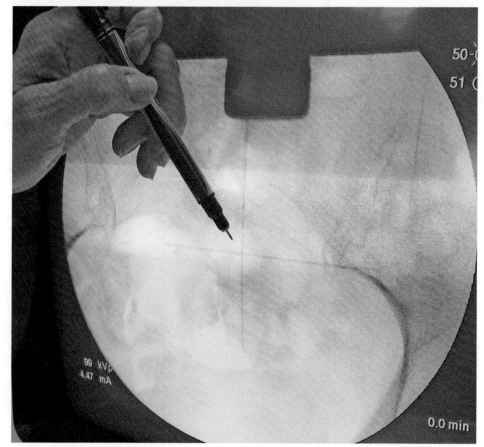

3. *S3 location.* Using fluoroscopy, the approximate location of the S3 spinal foramen is identified and marked at the skin level. Identification of S3 location is most commonly accomplished using a technique known as the crosshair technique. This method uses two spinal needles placed at right angles to each other to form a cruciform configuration using fluoroscopic guidance. The vertical needle is placed over the midline of the patient's spine. The horizontal needle is placed on a line formed by the ischial spines (Figure 11-7).

The S3 foramen is one fingerbreadth (1.5 to 2 cm) away from the cross junction of the needles.

4. *Foramen needle insertion.* A 20-gauge foramen needle is inserted at a 60-degree angle to the skin approximately 2 cm cranial to the actual location of the S3 foramen and directed caudally into the S3 foramen (Figure 11-8). Correct placement is confirmed by fluoroscopy (Figure 11-9). An electrical stimulus

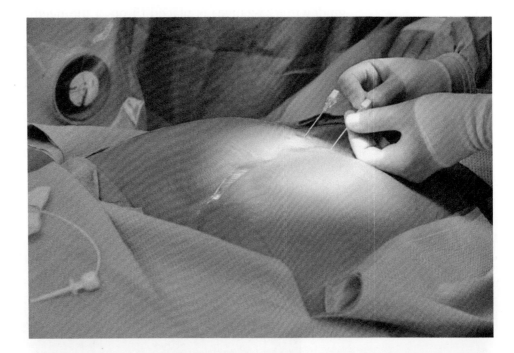

Figure 11-8 Placement of the foramen needle. The needle is inserted at an approximately 60-degree angle relative to the skin, approximately 2 cm cranial to the location of the sacral foramen.

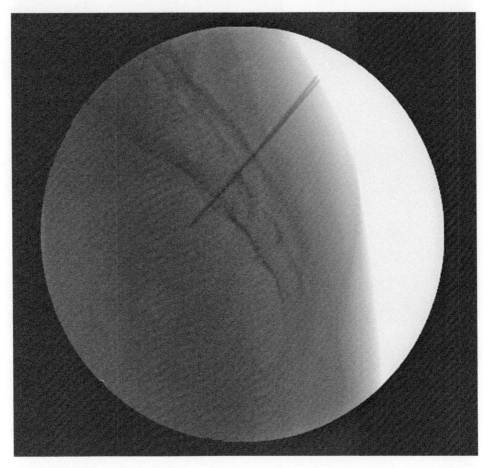

Figure 11-9 Fluoroscopic image of the foramen needle inserted into S3 foramen.

is applied to the foraminal needle via an external generator, and the pelvic floor and gluteal region and foot are examined for appropriate motor responses, which include a "bellows" response of the pelvic floor and ipsilateral great toe plantar flexion for S3 (see Table 11-1 and Figure 11-3). Bilateral foraminal needles can be placed to assess for the best response on each side.

5. *Lead introducer sheath placement.* When the S3 foramen is localized with the foramen needle, the inner stylet of the needle is removed, and a directional guidewire (23-gauge) is placed through the needle lumen and the needle is removed leaving the wire in place. A scalpel is used to incise the skin along the wire, and an introducer (composed of a 16-gauge dilator nestled in a 14-gauge introducer sheath) is passed over the wire to an appropriate depth of insertion determined by lateral fluoroscopy (Figure 11-10). Radiopaque markings on the introducer (one at the dilator tip and one at the introducer sheath tip) allow for accurate positioning of the device within the S3 foramen (Figure 11-11, *A*). The introducer sheath marking should be at the level of the ventral S3 foramen and the dilator tip marking just beyond. The introducer wire and dilator are removed, leaving the introducer sheath behind (Figure 11-11, *B*).

Figure 11-10 The lead introducer is inserted over the guidewire.

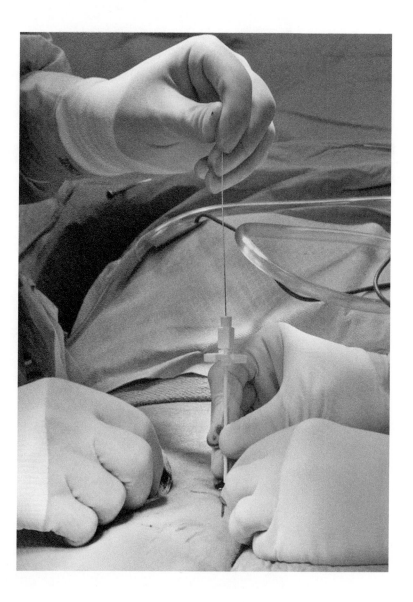

Figure 11-11 A, Fluoroscopic image of introducer inserted over the guidewire. The tip of the introducer should be just beyond to the ventral aspect of the S3 foramen. **B,** The introducer sheath remains in place after the guidewire and dilator have been removed.

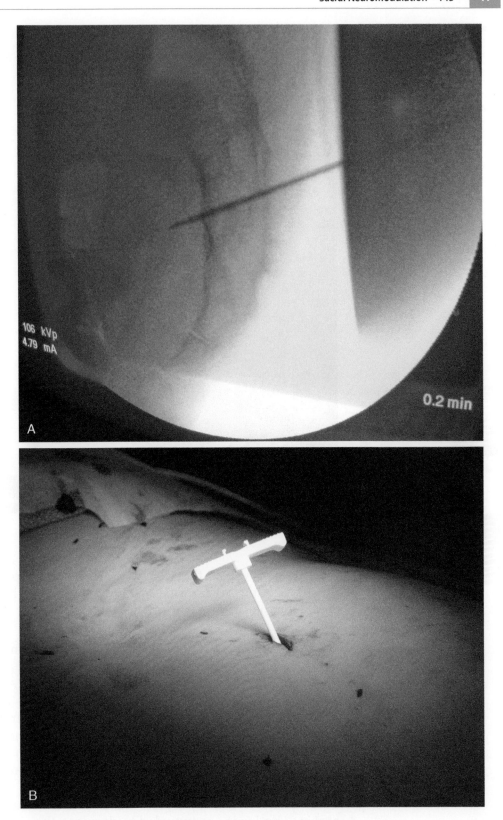

6. *Tined lead placement.* The tined lead is inserted into the sheath and positioned so that the electrical contact point No. 1 is straddling the ventral S3 foramen (Figure 11-12). The introducer sheath is slightly withdrawn, exposing the lead contact points without deploying the tined plastic projections. A white mark on the lead identifies the appropriate distance to withdraw the sheath. Electrical stimulation confirms the positioning of the lead at the

Figure 11-12 Fluoroscopic image of tined lead placement, lateral view. The lead is inserted until the electrical contact point No. 1 is straddling the ventral aspect of the S3 foramen.

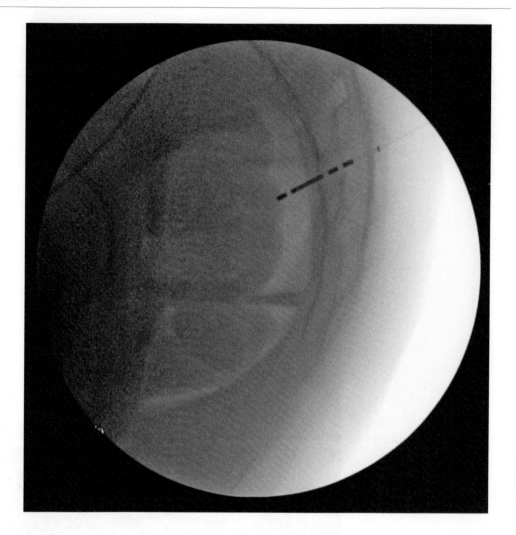

appropriate level; all four positions are tested for proper motor and sensory functions. After satisfactory positioning, the sheath is completely removed, deploying the tined plastic projections that anchor the lead to the surrounding soft tissue (Figure 11-13).

7. *Tunneling of lead.* A 3-cm skin incision is made in the contralateral upper buttocks, and a small subcutaneous pocket is created (Figure 11-14). This pocket is the future implantation site for the IPG. A tunneling trocar device is used to pass the stimulation lead into the IPG pocket (Figure 11-15). A bladed, tunneling trocar is passed subcutaneously from the site of percutaneous lead placement to the subcutaneous pocket; the bladed end is removed; the lead is passed through the remaining plastic sheath or tunneler; and the sheath is removed (Figure 11-16). A temporary, external lead extension is connected to the stimulation lead within the IPG pocket, and the external extension is tunneled further to exit the skin superolaterally to the IPG pocket. The leads are tunneled to decrease the risk of infection to the IPG device with externalized wires.

8. *Wound closure.* The redundant lead wire and connection covers are buried in the subcutaneous pocket previously developed, and the subcutaneous tissue and overlying skin are closed with absorbable sutures. The percutaneous tined lead insertion site is also closed with simple interrupted absorbable sutures (Figure 11-17).

Figure 11-13 Fluoroscopic image of tine lead, anterior-posterior view. When properly deployed, the lead demonstrates a slight lateral curve, conforming to the course of the S3 nerve root.

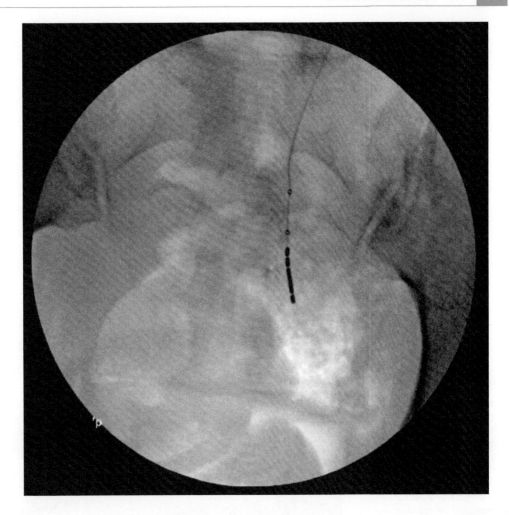

Figure 11-14 Incision and creation of subcutaneous pouch. A 3- to 4-cm incision in the contralateral upper buttocks is made and a subcutaneous pocket is developed at the future implantation site of the IPG.

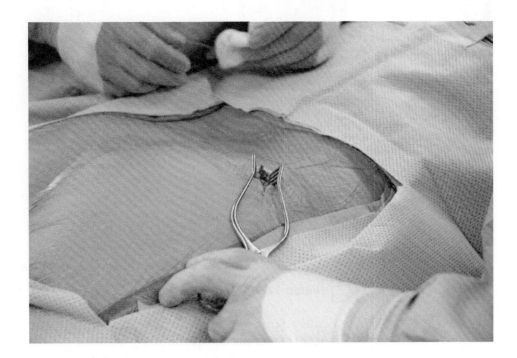

Figure 11-15 Tunneling device. The sharp pointed tunneling trocar device is used to tunnel the stimulation lead to the IPG pocket.

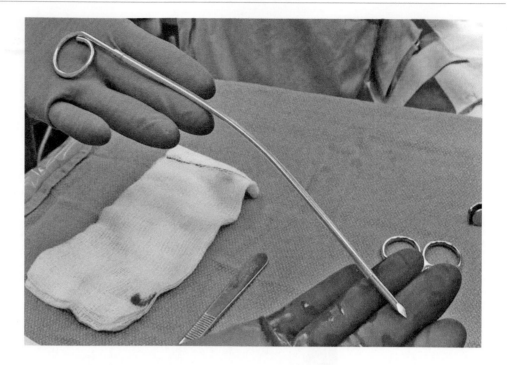

Figure 11-16 A bladed, tunneling trocar is passed subcutaneously from the site of percutaneous lead placement to the subcutaneous pocket; the bladed end is removed; the lead is passed through the remaining plastic sheath or tunneler; and the sheath is removed.

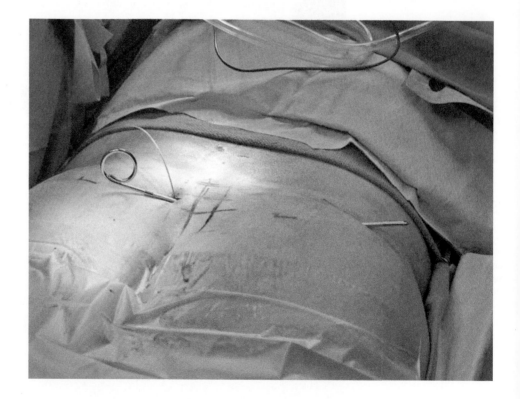

Implantable Pulse Generator Implantation, Second Stage

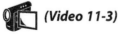 *(Video 11-3)*

1. *Anesthesia and patient positioning.* IPG implantation proceeds with the same anesthesia and patient positioning used for the first stage, as described previously. The skin area is sterilely cleansed, including the externalized, temporary lead, which is removed during this stage.

Figure 11-17 Completed stage 1. A temporary, external lead extension is attached to the lead; the connection is buried in the IPG pocket; and the external end is tunneled further laterally to exit superolaterally to the IPG pocket site.

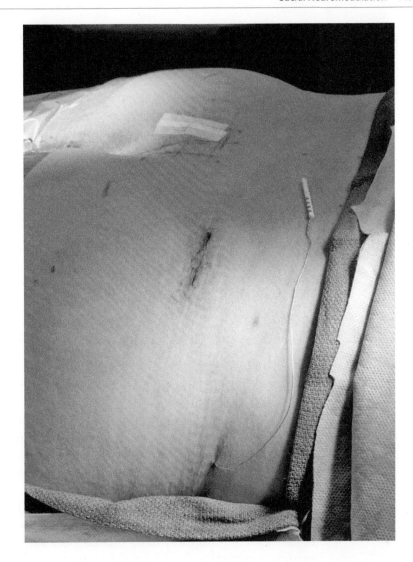

2. *IPG implantation.* The previous 3-cm incision over the buttocks is opened, and the buried electrical connection is exposed. The external lead extension is removed, and the subcutaneous pocket is enlarged to accommodate the IPG. The IPG is connected to the tined stimulation lead (using a hexagonal wrench with clockwise tightening until two audible clicks are heard), and the IPG is buried in the subcutaneous pocket (Figure 11-18). The skin incision is closed in a typical fashion.

Outcomes and Complications

Responses to SNM are variable, but most studies report an overall success rate (defined as >50% improvement in symptoms) of approximately 70% for patients with urgency, frequency, or urge incontinence (Bosch 2010; Siddiqui et al., 2010). For many patients, outcomes are durable for more than 5 years (Bosch 2010; Siegel et al., 2000). In a review of randomized controlled trials and case series, 80% of patients in the clinical trials achieved continence or greater than 50% improvement, and 67% of patients in the case series achieved similar results (Brazzelli et al., 2006). Results persisted over 3 to 5 years in these studies. However, despite widespread adoption of SNM, relatively few high-quality clinical studies are available to support these outcomes. A Cochrane

Figure 11-18 IPG implantation. During the second stage of implantation, the incision over the IPG site is made, and the tined lead–extension lead connection is disconnected. An IPG device is connected to the tined stimulation lead and inserted into the subcutaneous pocket. The overlying skin is closed with absorbable sutures.

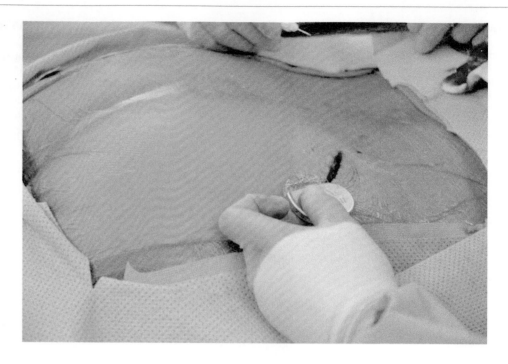

review identified only eight published studies from which data could not be pooled for meta-analysis (Herbison and Arnold 2009). Nevertheless, SNM is recommended as a second-line therapy for treatment of refractory overactive bladder and urge urinary incontinence (Abrams et al., 2010).

Few complications are seen with SNM; the complications generally relate to lead migration and loss of clinical benefit, device malfunction, or infection (Brazzelli et al., 2006; Chartier-Kastler 2008; Apostolidis 2011). Infection rates have been reported to be less than 5%. Revision rates usually for device malfunction are approximately 20%. Lead migration is one of the most common reasons for stimulation loss; this can be determined clinically with failure to restore stimulation despite reprogramming. For lead migration and device malfunction, a revision procedure, in which the lead or the IPG or both can be removed and reinserted, can restore previous effect levels. For infection, prompt surgical removal is warranted; a new device can be inserted at a later date. The safety and efficacy of SNM implants have not been established for use with magnetic resonance imaging, and patients who may require future or repeated magnetic resonance imaging studies should not undergo SNM implantation. Current IPG duration is estimated to be 5 to 7 years, depending on usage parameters. Device interrogation and frequent reprogramming are critical to therapy success and require outpatient infrastructure to support frequent use of these modulations to optimize therapy (Amend et al., 2011b).

Suggested Readings

Abrams P, Andersson KE, Birder L, et al.; Members of Committees; Fourth International Consultation. Fourth International Consultation on Incontinence Recommendations of the International Scientific Committee: evaluation and treatment of urinary incontinence, pelvic organ prolapse, and fecal incontinence. *Neurourol Urodyn.* 2010;29:213-240.

Amend B, Khalil M, Kessler TM, Sievert KD. How does sacral modulation work best? Placement and programming techniques to maximize efficacy. *Curr Urol Rep.* 2011a;12:327-335.

Amend B, Matzel KE, Abrams P, et al. How does neuromodulation work? *Neurourol Urodyn.* 2011b;30:762-765.

Apostolidis A. Neuromodulation for intractable OAB. *Neurourol Urodyn.* 2011;30:766-770.

Bosch JL. An update on sacral neuromodulation: where do we stand with this in the management of lower urinary tract dysfunction in 2010? *BJU Int.* 2010;106:1432-1442.

Brazzelli M, Murray A, Fraser C. Efficacy and safety of sacral nerve stimulation for urinary urge incontinence: a systematic review. *J Urol*. 2006;175(3 Pt 1):835-841.

Cameron AP, Anger JT, Madison R, Saigal CS, Clemens JQ. Urologic Diseases in America Project. National trends in the usage and success of sacral nerve test stimulation. *J Urol*. 2011;185:970-975.

Chartier-Kastler E. Sacral neuromodulation for treating the symptoms of overactive bladder syndrome and non-obstructive urinary retention: >10 years of clinical experience. *BJU Int*. 2008;101:417-423.

Herbison GP, Arnold EP. Sacral neuromodulation with implanted devices for urinary storage and voiding dysfunction in adults. *Cochrane Database Syst Rev*. 2009;(2):CD004202.

Leong RK, De Wachter SG, Nieman FH, de Bie RA, van Kerrebroeck PE. PNE versus 1st stage tined lead procedure: a direct comparison to select the most sensitive test method to identify patients suitable for sacral neuromodulation therapy. *Neurourol Urodyn*. 2011a;30:1249-1252.

Leong RK, De Wachter SG, van Kerrebroeck PE. Current information on sacral neuromodulation and botulinum toxin treatment for refractory idiopathic overactive bladder syndrome: a review. *Urol Int*. 2010;84:245-253.

Leong RK, Marcelissen TA, Nieman FH, De Bie RA, Van Kerrebroeck PE, De Wachter SG. Satisfaction and patient experience with sacral neuromodulation: results of a single center sample survey. *J Urol*. 2011b;185:588-592.

Marcelissen T, Leong R, Serroyen J, van Kerrebroeck P, de Wachter S. Is the screening method of sacral neuromodulation a prognostic factor for long-term success? *J Urol*. 2011;185:583-587.

Marcelissen TA, Leong RK, de Bie RA, van Kerrebroeck PE, de Wachter SG. Long-term results of sacral neuromodulation with the tined lead procedure. *J Urol*. 2010;184:1997-2000.

Occhino JA, Siegel SW. Sacral nerve modulation in overactive bladder. *Curr Urol Rep*. 2010;11:348-352.

Siddiqui NY, Wu JM, Amundsen CL. Efficacy and adverse events of sacral nerve stimulation for overactive bladder: a systematic review. *Neurourol Urodyn*. 2010;29(Suppl 1):S18-S23.

Siegel SW, Catanzaro F, Dijkema HE, et al. Long-term results of a multicenter study on sacral nerve stimulation for treatment of urinary urge incontinence, urgency-frequency, and retention. *Urology*. 2000;56(6 Suppl 1):87-91.

Botulinum Toxin Injection Therapy

W. Stuart Reynolds, M.D.
Melissa R. Kaufman, M.D.
Roger Dmochowski, M.D.

 Video

12-1 Technique of Intravesical
Injection of Botulinum Toxin

Introduction

Botulinum toxin (BoTN) is the most potent toxin known in the world. Through its neuromodulatory and paralytic mechanism, BoTN has been applied to facial cosmesis, muscle and neurologic spasticity, and migraine headaches. BoTN use for the treatment of voiding dysfunction has increased over the past several years and has had profound effects on patients with neurogenic bladder dysfunction and idiopathic detrusor overactivity (i.e., overactive bladder) when medical therapies fail. BoTN is easy to use and is generally well tolerated by the patient, with the benefits usually outweighing the adverse events. At the present time, BoTN is approved by the U.S. Food and Drug Administration (FDA) for use in the genitourinary system for neurogenic bladder, and FDA approval for idiopathic detrusor overactivity is expected in the near future.

Mechanism of Action

Depending on the serotype of the organism, *Clostridium botulinum,* seven distinct BoTNs can be produced by the bacterium (types A, B, C1, D, E, F, and G), all with similar mechanisms of action. At the present time, only BoTN A (Botox [Allergan, Irvine, CA] or Dysport [Medicis, Scottsdale, AZ]) and BoTN B (Myobloc or Neurobloc [Solstice Neuroscience, Louisville, KY]) are commercially available for clinical use. BoTN acts by cleaving a specific site (specific to each BoTN serotype) of a protein complex (soluble *N*-ethylmaleimide-sensitive fusion protein attachment protein receptor [SNARE] complex) responsible for exocytosis of neurotransmitter vesicles from the neuron. In the case of BoTN A, the most well-studied toxin subtype, the specific substrate is the synaptosomal associated protein of 25 kD (SNAP-25), a component of SNARE complex, which results in the inhibition of synaptic release of acetylcholine from the peripheral motor neuron end plate at the neuromuscular junction and ensuing muscle paralysis (Figure 12-1). More recent experience also suggests toxin effect on neurotransmitters related to sensory (afferent) function in the lower urinary tract.

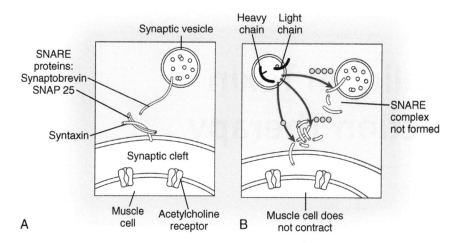

Figure 12-1 Mechanism of action of BoTN. **A,** In normal neurotransmitter release at the neuromuscular junction, the synaptic fusion complex comprising the SNARE proteins mediates synaptic vesicle fusion to the terminal membrane and acetylcholine exocytosis. **B,** In the presence of BoTN, which cleaves various SNARE proteins at sites specific to BoTN serotypes, the SNARE complex cannot form, and vesicle fusion and exocytosis is inhibited.

(From Koman LA, ed. Wake Forest University School of Medicine Orthopaedic Manual. Winston-Salem, NC: Orthopaedic Press; 2001.)

At therapeutic doses of 100 to 300 units, BoTN A induces paralysis in the detrusor muscle. However, BoTN A may additionally inhibit sensory nerve activity directly and modulate bladder sensory transmission to the central nervous system. In the cases of bladder overactivity (both neurogenic and idiopathic) and in bladder compliance abnormalities, both mechanisms of action are exploited.

BoTN A specifically is a noncompetitive agonist, and as such the effects are irreversible, yet also temporary as well. After administration of BoTN A, neuromuscular function is regained primarily through a process of motor neuron end plate regeneration and sprouting of the distal motor nerve. The duration of the effect is variable, but in the bladder, the clinical response to BoTN A injections lasts approximately 6 months.

The most common adverse event is increased post-void residual volume, which can occur in 10% to 20% of patients undergoing injection. Catheterization may be required, and secondary urinary tract infection may ensue. More recent changes in BoTN A labeling, in response to systemic effects associated with toxin use in skeletal muscle, include warnings regarding systemic absorption of toxin and respiratory effects resulting from disseminated toxin effects.

Case Scenario

 (Video 12-1)

A 59-year-old woman has had severe urge incontinence requiring multiple pads per day for more than 3 years. She is neurologically intact with no other significant morbidities. Physical examination is normal, and urinalysis and cytology are negative. She received two different antimuscarinic agents, each for 1 month, with dose escalation being used. She had no significant reduction in symptoms despite medication combination and optimizing behavioral therapy. Urodynamics reveals a maximum bladder capacity of 175 mL, with detrusor overactivity occurring at 100 mL with incontinence. There is no evidence of obstructed voiding, and minimal post-void residual is noted. Diagnostic cystoscopy is unremarkable. It is thought that this patient would be a good candidate for either neuromodulation or BoTN A injections. After risks and benefits of each of these therapies are discussed in great detail, the patient elects to proceed with BoTN A injections.

Botulinum Toxin Bladder Injection Technique

There is no standardized technique or approach to bladder injections of BoTN; a wide range of doses have been used, and many different injection templates have been followed. Generally, BoTN can be injected in the detrusor under direct cystoscopic guidance, with local or general anesthesia. A standard rigid or flexible cystourethroscope is used with a 23-gauge injection needle for toxin delivery. The effects of BoTN injection are apparent with symptom improvements noted within the first 7 to 10 days after injection. The therapeutic effects usually resolve after approximately 6 months, although after sequential injections (third or more) the beneficial effects may last longer (up to 9 months).

Because most clinical experience involves the use of BoTN A serotype, this discussion focuses on this toxin subtype. Dosing of BoTN is defined by units of biologic activity and are neither interchangeable nor directly comparable with other BoTN types. BoTN A is supplied in 100-unit and 200-unit vials as a desiccated powder (Figure 12-2), which is reconstituted immediately before injection with injectable grade, preservative-free normal saline. Dosing protocols vary, and 50 to 300 units may be injected at a single session. Depending on the desired concentration of injection solution, 10 mL of injectable saline is used to dissolve each vial of BoTN A, and the solution is drawn up in appropriately sized syringes. Typically, injection of BoTN proceeds with 10 to 30 submucosal injection sites spread across the base and posterior wall of the bladder, including or not including the trigone, and injection of 0.1 to 1 mL each of BoTN solution, depending on the concentration (approximately 10 units per injection) (Figure 12-3).

1. *Patient position.* The patient is positioned in a standard dorsal lithotomy position and prepared sterilely in a fashion usual for cystoscopy. Periprocedural antibiotics are administered.

2. *Analgesia.* Local anesthetic is used, with 2% lidocaine jelly injected intraurethrally followed by intravesical instillation of 100 mL of 2% lidocaine solution. Dwell time for the solution should be at least 20 minutes.

3. *BoTN solution reconstitution.* The desiccated powder is reconstituted with preservative-free, injectable grade 0.9% saline, as discussed previously.

4. *Cystoscopy.* Cystourethroscopy is performed initially. In addition to noting any abnormality within the bladder, understanding the size and

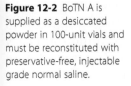

Figure 12-2 BoTN A is supplied as a desiccated powder in 100-unit vials and must be reconstituted with preservative-free, injectable grade normal saline.

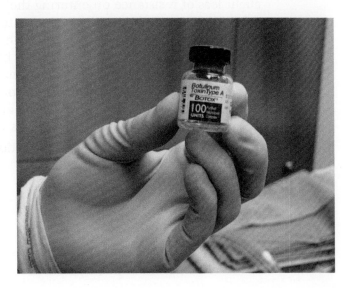

Figure 12-3 Injection techniques vary, and many different injection templates have been described. A typical template involves 20 to 30 bladder injections spread over the posterior aspect of the bladder and dome and may or may not include the bladder trigone.

(From Kim DK, Thomas CA, Smith C, Chancellor MB. The case for bladder botulinum toxin application. Urol Clin North Am. *2006;33:503-510.)*

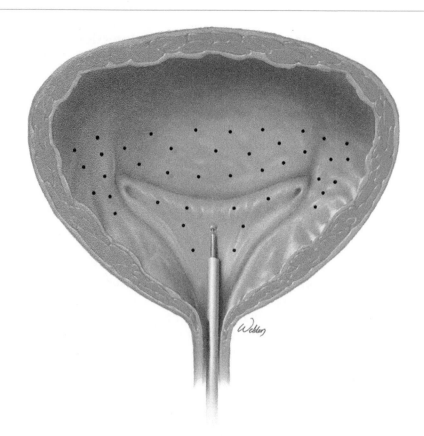

configuration of the bladder helps in planning the spacing of BoTN injections so as to cover as much of the bladder as possible. Ideally, approximately 10 to 30 injections should be used to deliver the BoTN, and the required volume should be taken into consideration during reconstitution (see Figure 12-3). The trigone is not injected.

5. *BoTN injection.* With the cystoscope in the bladder, the 23-gauge needle (with BoTN-containing syringe attached) is advanced out of the tip of the scope and directed toward the desired injection location (Figure 12-4). Care should be taken to avoid inserting the needle through a visible blood vessel in the bladder mucosa because this can lead to bothersome bleeding. The needle is advanced into the submucosa approximately 0.5 cm; typically, there is a slight loss of resistance on entering the mucosa. Once positioned, the BoTN solution is gently injected, approximately 0.5 to 1 mL, depending on concentration (Figure 12-5). Injecting at the appropriate depth is important to avoid extravasating BoTN through the bladder wall or depositing the BoTN too superficially within the bladder mucosa. Ideally, injecting the solution raises the overlying mucosa only minimally, avoiding large blebs on the mucosal surface. After delivery, the needle is withdrawn and repositioned at the next location, and the process is repeated.

6. The bladder is drained at the completion of toxin delivery and postprocedural instructions are given.

Outcomes and Complications

Of patients treated for overactive bladder symptoms with BoTN A bladder injection, 60% to 80% show improvements in symptoms. Approximately 70% of

Figure 12-4 A, A 22F rigid injection cystoscope with **(B)** a 22-gauge injection needle is used to injected BoTNA. Alternatively, a flexible cystoscope and corresponding injection needle can be used.

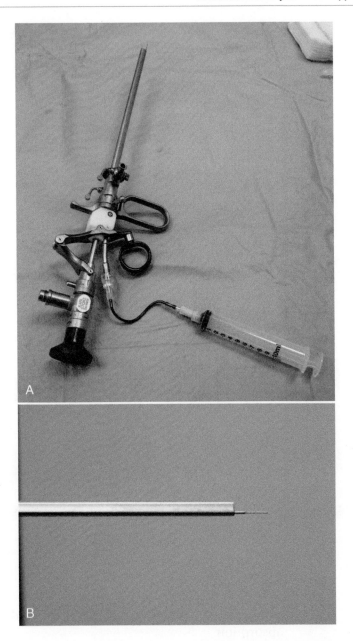

patients with neurogenic detrusor abnormalities have improvement. Efficacy is generally limited to 6 months because the effects abate as noted previously. Repeat injection can be performed with similar efficacy anticipated.

Controversy exists regarding whether or not the bladder trigone should be included in the injection template because there has been some theoretical concern of inducing vesicoureteral reflux by injecting near the ureteral orifices. This concern has not been substantiated clinically. Because the trigone is thought to be densely innervated, many clinicians regularly include it in the template.

The major adverse event related to BoTN bladder injection is increased post-void residual volume, which has been reported to occur approximately 10% to 20% of the time. Patients should be counseled regarding intermittent self-catheterization in the event that retention ensues. Retention is typically transient and resolves with time (usually ≤1 month). Minor complications of the procedure include transient dysuria, hematuria, and occasional urinary tract infection. More worrisome are rare reports of generalized weakness, malaise,

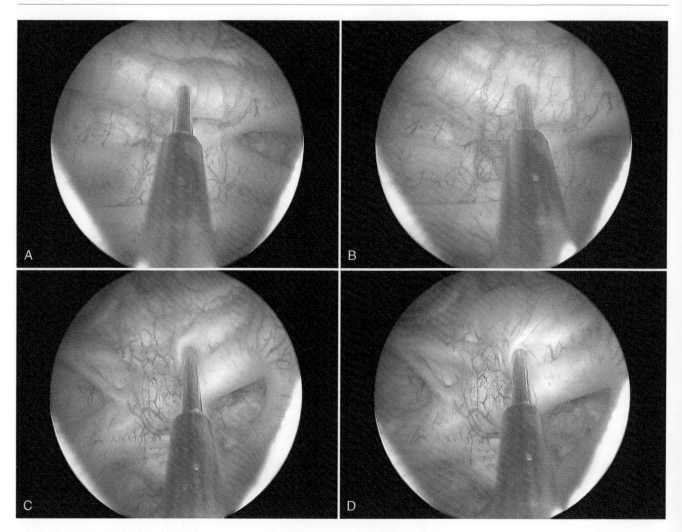

Figure 12-5 A-D, To achieve the proper depth of injection, the needle should be inserted through the mucosa **(A** and **C)**, typically with a slight "popping" feel, and the injected material should raise the overlying mucosa minimally, as demonstrated in the images by the "filling" of the areas between bladder trabeculae **(B** and **D)**.

and muscle weakness, possibly secondary to systemic effects of BoTN absorption.

Generally, the effect of BoTN A injection diminishes with time and abates by approximately 6 months after treatment. At this time, symptoms generally redevelop, and repeated injection is necessary to recoup any clinical benefit previously seen. With appropriate counseling, patients often are aware of this development and seek evaluation when they perceive the benefits are wearing off.

BoTN effect may be minimized in the presence of acute urinary tract infection, and urinary tract infection should be excluded before injection. Concomitant aminoglycoside administration at the time of toxin injection may obviate BoTN effect and should be avoided.

Injection depth should be optimized (entire needle point placed into detrusor) to optimize therapy. Some patients may experience a variability in response over sequential injections (the magnitude of efficacy effect may vary between injections), and individuals undergoing repeat injections should be made aware of this possibility.

Increased urinary residual volume and urinary retention are the most common complications. This outcome can be mitigated by initial dosing at low levels with gradual increase of toxin dose over time balancing effect and side effects to determine optimal individual dose magnitude.

Conclusion

With the FDA approval of BoTN for neurogenic causes of detrusor overactivity and likely approval for idiopathic detrusor overactivity in the near future, the authors believe this therapy will be a good addition to the armamentarium of therapies available for this common, very distressing problem.

Suggested Readings

Abdel-Meguid TA. Botulinum toxin-A injections into neurogenic overactive bladder—to include or exclude the trigone? A prospective, randomized, controlled trial. *J Urol.* 2010;184:2423-2428.

Anger JT, Weinberg A, Suttorp MJ, Litwin MS, Shekelle PG. Outcomes of intravesical botulinum toxin for idiopathic overactive bladder symptoms: a systematic review of the literature. *J Urol.* 2010;183: 2258-2264.

Dmochowski R, Chapple C, Nitti VW, et al. Efficacy and safety of onabotulinumtoxinA for idiopathic overactive bladder: a double-blind, placebo controlled, randomized, dose ranging trial. *J Urol.* 2010; 184:2416-2422.

Kuo HC, Liao CH, Chung SD. Adverse events of intravesical botulinum toxin A injections for idiopathic detrusor overactivity: risk factors and influence on treatment outcome. *Eur Urol.* 2010;58:919-926.

Leong RK, de Wachter SG, Joore MA, van Kerrebroeck PE. Cost-effectiveness analysis of sacral neuro-modulation and botulinum toxin A treatment for patients with idiopathic overactive bladder. *BJU Int.* 2011;108:558-564.

Mehnert U, Birzele J, Reuter K, Schurch B. The effect of botulinum toxin type A on overactive bladder symptoms in patients with multiple sclerosis: a pilot study. *J Urol.* 2010;184:1011-1016.

Bladder Augmentation

13

W. Stuart Reynolds, M.D.
Melissa R. Kaufman, M.D.
Roger Dmochowski, M.D.

 Video

13-1 Technique for Bladder
Augmentation (Example 1)

13-2 Technique for Bladder
Augmentation (Example 2)

Introduction

When less invasive measures have failed in the treatment of bladder storage (phasic contraction and compliance) abnormalities, the most aggressive management option is augmentation cystoplasty. The goal of bladder augmentation is to create a large-capacity, low-pressure (i.e., high compliance) reservoir for urine storage. Larger volumes of urine may be stored for longer periods, which is beneficial for continence, while the detrusor pressure remains low, protecting the upper urinary system and kidneys from dysfunction and ultimately renal failure. This goal is generally achieved at the cost of efficient bladder emptying, and at least one third of patients are dependent on intermittent catheterization for bladder drainage after augmentation.

Many different techniques have been developed for augmentation cystoplasty using various tissues for augmentation, including segments of detubularized large and small intestine (ileocystoplasty, cecocystoplasty, sigmoid cystoplasty, and gastrocystoplasty), dilated ureter (ureteroplasty), autoaugmentation (removal of the overlying detrusor muscle of the dome of the bladder), and, more recently, biologic substitutes employing bioengineered tissue. The most common procedure involves the use of small intestine, specifically the ileum.

If the native urethra is to be abandoned, a cutaneous catheterizable stoma can be created to allow for efficient intermittent catheterization and emptying. Direct obstructive closure of the bladder neck can be achieved surgically with ablation (via transection and oversewing of the bladder outlet) or functionally with a compressive suburethral sling.

Case Scenario

 (Video 13-1)

A 62-year-old woman who has had urge incontinence and bothersome urinary frequency (12 voids per 24 hours) for more than 3 years, without known neurologic disease or other significant morbidities, with a normal physical examination, and negative urinalysis and cytology requests therapy for her symptoms. She has received two different antimuscarinic agents, each for 1 month, with dose escalation being used and with no significant reduction in symptoms despite medication combination with optimized behavioral therapy. Percutaneous tibial stimulation was performed with some short-term success, after which botulinum toxin injections (100 units) were attempted without significant benefit. Urodynamics reveals a bladder capacity of 180 mL, with detrusor overactivity occurring at 30 mL, 60 mL, and 180 mL with incontinence and no evidence of obstructed voiding and minimal post-void residual. Diagnostic cystoscopy is unremarkable. Based on the severity of the situation and the fact that objective testing noted very low-capacity, high-pressure detrusor overactivity with very poor compliance, it is decided to proceed with an augmentation cystoplasty.

Surgical Technique

The general procedure for augmentation ileocystoplasty is illustrated in Figure 13-1.

1. The patient is typically positioned supine on the operating room table or in the low lithotomy position with legs in stirrups. Surgical skin preparation should include the abdomen, perineum, and genitalia (to provide access to the urethral catheter for bladder volume manipulation with saline and controlled drainage during detrusor resection and bowel-to-bladder anastomosis).

2. The operation proceeds via a standard lower midline laparotomy incision. A midline incision is made from the pubis to the umbilicus and carried down through the anterior abdominal fascia, splitting the rectus muscles and opening the transversalis fascia and peritoneum.

3. The bladder is prepared with a sagittal incision almost completely bivalving the bladder, extending from 3 cm above the bladder neck anteriorly to 2 cm above the trigone posteriorly (Figure 13-2). Filling the bladder with saline before incising the detrusor can facilitate maintaining a sagittal plane of incision.

4. To prepare bowel segment to be used for augmentation, the terminal ileum is identified, and a segment of ileum approximately 20 to 40 cm in length is isolated 15 cm or more proximal to the ileocecal valve. Care is taken to divide the mesentery so as to preserve blood supply to both the isolated ileal segment and the limbs of the bowel anastomosis (Figure 13-3, *A*). Bowel division and subsequent anastomosis can be performed either with hand-sewn sutures or with bowel anastomotic staplers (Figure 13-3, *B*).

5. The isolated section of ileum is detubularized longitudinally along its anti-mesenteric border using electrocautery (Figure 13-4). Typically, the bowel is reconfigured in either a "U" shape or an "S" shape by folding the bowel and suturing the inner edges with full-thickness, running 2-0 or 3-0 absorbable polydioxanone suture (see Figure 13-4).

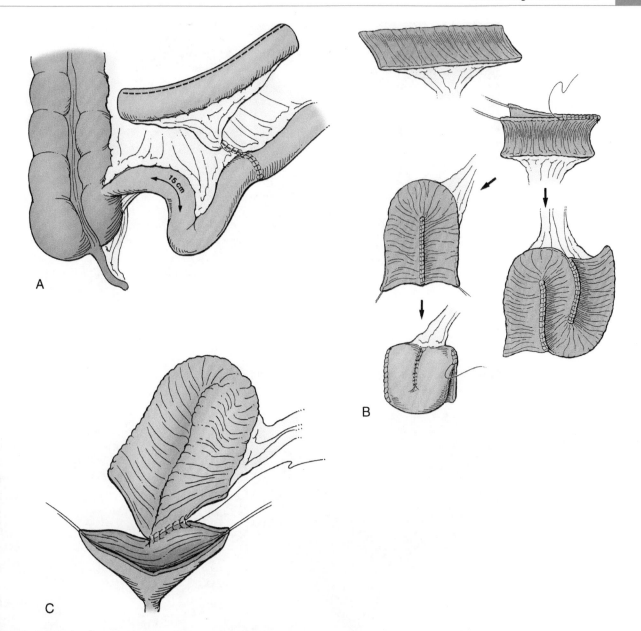

Figure 13-1 A, Augmentation ileal cystoplasty entails isolating a segment of distal ileum (while preserving the terminal ileum and ileocecal valve). **B,** Opening the segment longitudinally, reconfiguring the ileal patch. **C,** Anastomosing the reconfigured patch to a sagittally bivalved bladder.

(From Wein AJ, et al., eds. Campbell-Walsh Urology, ed 10. Philadelphia: Saunders; 2012.)

6. The reconfigured bowel is anastomosed to the bivalved bladder, starting at the posterior margin, with running 2-0 or 3-0 absorbable suture, along each of the sagittally incised bladder edges (see Figure 13-4). Before complete closure, a suprapubic tube is placed, exiting through the native bladder wall, and a urethral catheter is placed. The bladder is irrigated with saline to confirm that it is watertight (Figure 13-5); a closed-suction drain is placed, and both drains are brought out through the skin in separate stab incisions. The abdominal wall is finally closed in customary fashion.

Postoperative Care and Considerations (Video 13-2 📹)

The suprapubic tube and urethral catheter are left in place for approximately 10 to 21 days, at which time a cystogram can be obtained to confirm that there

Figure 13-2 A, To prepare the bladder, a sagittal cystotomy is made in the dome of the bladder. **B** and **C,** The cystotomy is carried anteriorly to 3 cm above the bladder neck **(B)** and posteriorly to 2 cm above the trigonal ridge **(C)**. **D,** The prepared bladder is almost completely bivalved in the sagittal plane. The ureteral orifices are denoted by the *arrows*.

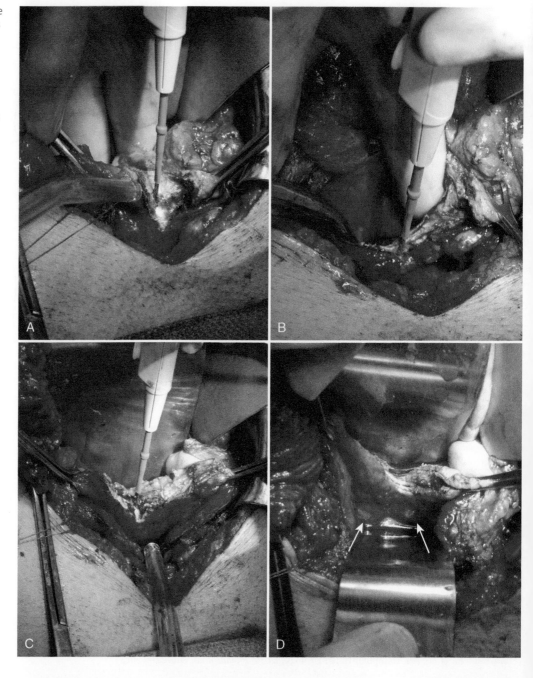

Figure 13-3 A, To isolate the bowel segment, the mesentery is divided so as to preserve blood supply to both the ileum segment and the eventual bowel anastomosis. **B,** Bowel division and reanastomosis may be formed with either a hand-sewn technique or a bowel anastomotic stapler, as pictured. A 3.8-mm straight gastrointestinal stapler is used to divide the ileum.

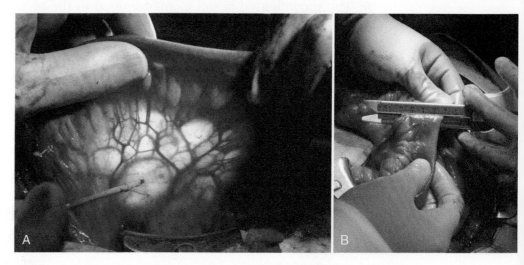

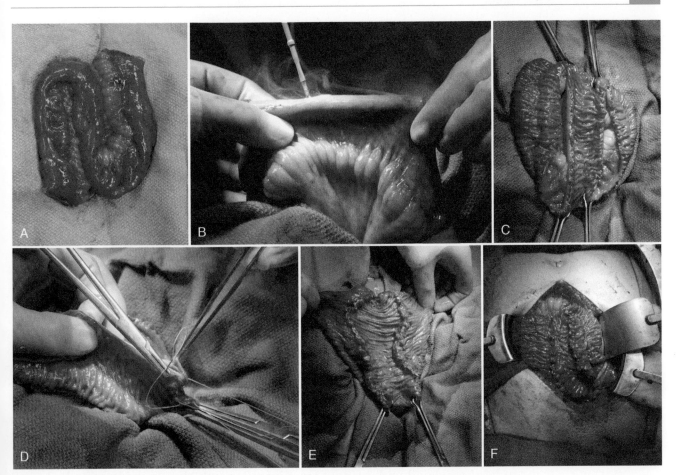

Figure 13-4 A, Typically, the bowel is reconfigured before anastomosing to the bladder to maximize spherical surface area; in this case, the bowel was arranged in an "S" shape. **B,** The bowel is incised longitudinally along the antimesentery border with electrocautery to detubularize the segment completely. **C,** The "S" configuration of the incised bowel before suturing is demonstrated. **D,** The two internal cut edges of the bowel are sutured longitudinally in a simple, running technique with 2-0 absorbable suture. **E,** The completely reconfigured ileal patch is shown aligned for anastomosis to the bladder. **F,** Beginning at the posterior apex of the bladder incision, the outer cut edges of the ileal patch and bivalved bladder are sutured in a single layer with 2-0 absorbable suture, progressing in an anterior fashion until the entire patch is anastomosed to the bladder, effectively "clamshelling" the ileal segment onto the dome of the bladder.

is no urinary extravasation. The urethral catheter is removed, the suprapubic tube is clamped, and the patient is taught clean intermittent catheterization. When the patient is comfortable with catheterization, the suprapubic tube can be removed. Typically, the patient is instructed to perform clean intermittent catheterization every 2 to 3 hours during the day and once or twice at night. The frequency of catheterizations can be decreased to every 4 hours. If the patient demonstrates the ability to empty completely, clean intermittent catheterization can be discontinued.

Follow-up after augmentation should include regular renal imaging (ultrasound, intravenous pyelogram, or renal scan) during the first year and subsequently at regular intervals to monitor for upper urinary tract changes. Additionally, serum electrolytes and creatinine levels should be monitored regularly during this time to screen for electrolyte and metabolic abnormalities. Because of the possibility of gut absorptive abnormalities caused by intestinal resection, an annual serum vitamin B_{12} level should also be obtained. Finally, because of the risk of tumor formation, surveillance should be performed with annual cystoscopy (beginning 5 years after surgery).

Figure 13-5 The completed ileal augmentation is shown and is filled with saline, confirming the closure is watertight. A suprapubic tube is placed before complete closure and brought out to the abdominal wall through a separate stab incision.

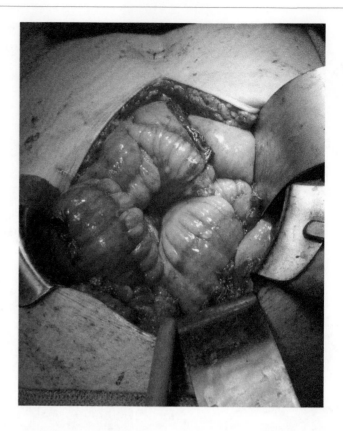

Bacteriuria is a common finding after augmentation, particularly in patients performing clean intermittent catheterization. However, it need not be treated unless associated with urinary tract infection, which is considered to be bacteriuria associated with symptoms of fever, suprapubic pain, hematuria, foul-smelling urine, incontinence, or increased mucus production. Antibiotic therapy should be organism-specific based on urinary culture results. Other complications of bladder augmentation are bladder stone formation, thought to be related to urease-splitting bacteria urinary tract infection, uncleared mucus, hypercalciuria, residual urine or bladder foreign bodies, overproduction of mucus, metabolic acidosis because of abnormal reabsorption of urinary ammonium, and idiopathic bladder perforation.

In patients undergoing augmentation cystoplasty, improvements in continence can be expected in more than three of four patients, with 50% or more being completely continent. Most reports suggest 70% improvement rates (improved and cured) in patients undergoing augmentation.

Conclusion

Augmentation cystoplasty has historically been used as salvage therapy for patients failing medical therapy for bladder storage abnormalities. With the advent of neuromodulation, rates of bladder augmentation have decreased substantially (Biers et al., 2011). The potential addition of botulinum toxin to the therapeutic paradigm may also affect the rates of augmentation. These effects are not untoward given the potential short-term and long-term consequences of augmentation as noted previously. Additionally, some evidence suggests that long-term quality of life in patients who have undergone augmentation is not as satisfactory as would be hoped. Enlightened informed consent is crucial before embarking on this intervention.

Mucus production can be problematic and should be managed with vitamin C and citrus products (to acidify the urine). Self-irrigation periodically with sterile water may also be helpful.

Abdominal pain in a patient after augmentation should be presumed to be representative of augment perforation, which should be excluded by urgent cystogram (fluoroscopy or computed tomography). Free fluid on computed tomography scan is consistent with this diagnosis and should warrant consideration of exploratory laparotomy.

Suggested Readings

Biers SM, Venn SN, Greenwell TJ. The past, present and future of augmentation cystoplasty. *BJU Int.* 2011;109:1280-1293.

Reyblat P, Ginsberg DA. Augmentation enterocystoplasty in overactive bladder: is there still a role? *Curr Urol Rep.* 2010;11:432-439.

Mixed and Recurrent Incontinence, Incontinence in Patients with Pelvic Organ Prolapse, and How Best to Avoid and Manage Complications: Case Discussions

14

Mickey Karram, M.D.
W. Stuart Reynolds, M.D.
Roger Dmochowski, M.D.

 Videos

Introduction

This chapter discusses the management of mixed and recurrent stress incontinence, the management of incontinence in conjunction with pelvic organ prolapse, and how best to avoid and manage intraoperative and postoperative complications that can occur when performing procedures to correct stress incontinence. These discussions are presented in a case presentation format. A video clip to demonstrate and illustrate the various complications accompanies most cases. Complications related to urinary retention and voiding dysfunction are not included in this chapter because they are discussed in Chapter 9.

Case 1: Mixed Incontinence

A 62-year-old woman presents with symptoms of severe incontinence. She describes her incontinence as being both stress and urge related. She wears numerous pads every day, and when asked whether she is more bothered by the stress or the urge component, she states they are equally bothersome. Initial attempts at nonsurgical management include antimuscarinic therapy, timed voiding, pelvic floor rehabilitation, and behavioral therapy. Although these modalities significantly improve the urge component of her leakage, she continues to complain of fairly severe stress incontinence and desires definitive therapy for this. Urodynamics testing notes readily demonstrable stress urinary incontinence (SUI) at a volume of 150 mL with leak point pressures of 80 cm H_2O. She has an uninhibited bladder contraction at a volume of 500 mL that is associated with a large volume leak. The patient gives consent for a transobturator sling fully understanding that the natural history of the urge component of her leakage was unpredictable. After the sling procedure, she has correction of SUI, but urge symptoms persist.

Discussion of Case

Mixed urinary incontinence (MUI) refers to the complaint of involuntary leakage associated with urgency and with increases in intra-abdominal pressure such as coughing and straining. More recent data and expert consensus support the selective use of anti-incontinence procedures to correct SUI in patients with mixed symptoms who have a significant SUI component (Dmochowski et al., 2010). Both retropubic and transobturator tape (TOT) midurethral slings (MUS) have been shown to have excellent cure rates of 85% to 97% for the stress component (Jain et al., 2011). Researchers have also analyzed the efficacy of MUS in treating the urge components and which factors predict better or worse outcomes. Several studies have compared efficacy of retropubic and TOT slings for the treatment of women with MUI. Gamble et al. (2008) reported 305 women with objective evidence of SUI and detrusor overactivity undergoing TOT, tension-free vaginal tape (TVT), SPARC (American Medical Systems, Minneapolis, MN), or biologic bladder neck sling procedures. Primary outcome was persistent detrusor overactivity at 3 months. Resolution of detrusor overactivity differed significantly between the groups with the best results after TOT slings (47%) followed by retropubic slings (37%) and bladder neck slings (14%) ($P > .001$). Subjective cure of urge incontinence was seen in 44% of the whole group. In contrast, a similar study by Botros et al. (2007) found no difference in resolution of detrusor overactivity 3 months after retropubic versus TOT slings. A large observational cohort by Lee et al. (2010b) studied 514 women with MUI and 754 women with SUI and urge symptoms (but no urge incontinence) who were treated with retropubic or TOT slings. At a mean follow-up of 50 months, there was resolution of urge incontinence in 67.7% and urge symptoms in 59.7%. Preoperative detrusor overactivity, which was objectively demonstrated on urodynamics testing, was a risk factor for persistent urge incontinence and urgency.

Some studies with longer follow-up have demonstrated less encouraging outcomes. Kulseng-Hanssen et al. (2008) reported on a series of 1113 patients with MUI at 38 months after TVT and found a subjective cure rate of 53.8%. When only patients with predominantly urge incontinence were considered, subjective cure rate was 38.4%; however, patient satisfaction was still 60%.

Patients with complaints of MUI are extremely challenging when contemplating surgical correction. At the present time, based on available literature, the authors prefer whenever possible to manage these patients with a TOT sling in contrast to a retropubic or single-incision sling. Patients need to be counseled and to understand fully that the outcome of the urge component of their leakage is unpredictable, and there is a possibility that it could persist or worsen after sling placement.

Case 2: Recurrent Stress Urinary Incontinence After Two Previous Unsuccessful Synthetic Midurethral Sling Procedures

 (Video 14-1)

A 38-year-old woman presents with dyspareunia and severe recurrent stress incontinence; she has received two previous synthetic MUS and an anterior trocar-based mesh kit for a cystocele. There is no evidence of mesh erosion into the anterior vaginal wall; however, significant pain is elicited on palpation of the middle of the anterior vaginal wall secondary to mesh shrinkage. Urodynamics confirms severe SUI secondary to intrinsic sphincter deficiency, and examination of the anterior vaginal wall notes minimal urethral mobility (Q-tip strain angle of 15 degrees). Cystoscopy is negative for any mesh erosion. The patient gives consent for excision of previously placed suburethral portions of the synthetic slings, with vaginal urethrolysis (in the hope of creating more urethral mobility) excision of mesh from the anterior vaginal wall, and placement of a rectus fascia pubovaginal sling under the proximal urethra.

During the removal of one of the synthetic slings, it became apparent that sling material was in the wall of the urethra. Sharp excision of the polypropylene from the wall of the urethra was required resulting in a urethrotomy; this was repaired in two layers ensuring that the lumen of the urethra was not constricted. Because there was an appropriate blood supply, no vascular pedicle was thought to be needed, and we proceeded with placement of the rectus fascia sling. Postoperatively, the patient had complete resolution of SUI and vaginal pain, but she developed de novo urgency and urge incontinence, which required antimuscarinic therapy and pelvic floor rehabilitation.

Discussion of Case

Evaluation and treatment of women with persistent or recurrent SUI after a previous incontinence procedure depend on the nature of the original treatment; the presence or absence of associated urgency, frequency, and voiding dysfunction; and the current state of the surrounding tissue. Approximately 10% to 20% of women undergoing a sling procedure have persistent or recurrent SUI. Objective data to guide the appropriate choice of a secondary surgical procedure are limited. Generally, women with persistent or recurrent SUI should undergo a thorough evaluation, which almost always includes urodynamics studies and endoscopic assessment. The operative notes from the original surgery should be obtained if at possible. Although there are no good studies currently evaluating the role of a repeat synthetic MUS after a failed synthetic MUS, the overall cure rates for repeat MUS have been shown to be lower than the cure rates for primary surgery. In uncontrolled case series, both retropubic and transobturator MUS have been shown to be effective salvage procedures at least in the short term. One large retrospective series suggested that retropubic MUS have a higher success rate than TOT MUS for patients with recurrent SUI. The authors have preferred to use retropubic MUS in patients who have failed TOT MUS. In patients who have failed single-incision MUS, TOT or retropubic MUS may be used. Sabaddel et al. reported good results with the use of retropubic TVT for recurrent SUI after failed TOT with overall cure and improvement rates of 86.4% at 12 months and 75% at 36 months.

In patients who have failed retropubic MUS, a repeat retropubic MUS and traditional pubovaginal sling are acceptable options. Although data are limited, the authors have also found retropubic MUS to be successful in patients with failed colposuspension with decreased bladder neck mobility. If the urethra is hypermobile, TOT MUS would also be a viable option. Finally, in patients who have a fixed urethra, are unstable, or are unwilling to undergo repeat surgery, paraurethral bulking can be considered (see Chapter 10).

Case 3: Stress Incontinence in Conjunction with Symptomatic Pelvic Organ Prolapse

A 71-year-old, para 3 woman presents with a primary complaint of pelvic pressure and tissue protrusion. She states that over the last 6 months she has felt a bulge of tissue that extends well beyond the opening of the vagina and has become very bothersome to her. She had a vaginal hysterectomy 30 years ago for irregular uterine bleeding. When asked about bladder function, she states that recently as the bulge has developed she has developed significant frequency and urgency and difficulty initiating her void. She denies any past history of SUI. On examination, she is noted to have significant anterior vaginal wall prolapse (stage 3) with point AA being +3 and AB being +6. She is also noted to have apical prolapse to the level of the hymen and a rectocele with a widened genital hiatus. She desires definitive therapy in the form of surgery for pelvic organ prolapse. Lower urinary tract assessment involves obtaining a post-void residual, which is noted to be 50 mL after voiding of 400 mL. An eyeball filling study notes a maximum capacity of 480 mL. The sign of stress incontinence cannot be demonstrated with the prolapse unreduced; however, when the prolapse is gently reduced with half of a bivalve speculum, obvious SUI is noted in the supine position with aggressive coughing. In view of these findings, the patient is scheduled for a TOT sling in conjunction with vaginal prolapse repair.

Discussion of Case

More than 50% of women who present with systematic pelvic organ prolapse complain of SUI symptoms, and 24% complain of symptoms of MUI. Present data indicate that women with pelvic organ prolapse and SUI who undergo surgery have lower rates of postoperative SUI if MUS procedure is performed concurrent with pelvic organ prolapse surgery. Both retropubic and transobturator MUS have been shown to be effective in this setting. Women undergoing pelvic organ prolapse surgery who have a history of SUI symptoms, demonstrate a positive stress test, or demonstrate a positive stress test with reduction of the prolapse probably should undergo a simultaneous MUS procedure at the time of the prolapse repair. We prefer to perform TOT MUS in older patients, patients with mixed symptoms, or patients with evidence of voiding dysfunction; however, in younger patients and patients with recurrent SUI, we prefer retropubic MUS. At the present time, some data indicate that women who undergo prolapse repair with synthetic mesh to correct anterior vaginal wall prolapse are at increased risk for either de novo development of SUI or persistent or worsening of pre-existing SUI. We usually perform retropubic MUS in these situations. It is hypothesized that the additional anatomic support provided by the placement of anterior vaginal mesh straightens the bladder neck and ultimately compromises the continence mechanism, although this is unclear. More data are required to support such a theory.

Case 4: Bladder Perforation at the Time of Retropubic Synthetic Midurethral Sling Procedure

 (Video 14-2)

A 57-year-old woman presents with recurrent SUI. She had a Burch colposuspension approximately 10 years ago. She remained continent until recently and now complains of numerous accidents on a daily basis that require protective clothing. On examination, she is noted to have a fairly well-supported bladder neck with a mild amount of urethral hypermobility (Q-tip straining angle of 25 degrees). Cystourethroscopy demonstrates a normal urethra and bladder with no evidence of any suture penetration or foreign body from the previous Burch procedure. Urodynamics studies note a stable detrusor to a maximum capacity of 445 mL. She easily demonstrates urodynamic stress incontinence at a volume of 150 mL with a Valsalva leak point pressure of 43 cm H_2O. After a detailed discussion, it is decided to proceed with retropubic synthetic MUS. During the procedure, there was evidence of perforation of the bladder bilaterally requiring a second passage of the retropubic needle on each side. Ultimately, the sling was placed in an appropriate location, and the patient was sent to the recovery room with a Foley catheter in place.

Discussion of Case

Bladder perforation at the time of retropubic synthetic sling placement occurs in approximately 3% to 5% of cases. The needle almost always perforates the bladder high up between the 1 o'clock and 3 o'clock position on the left side and the 9 o'clock and 11 o'clock position on the right side. The penetration usually occurs secondary to cephalad migration of the needle away from the back of the pubic bone. Because the site of penetration is usually high up in a nondependent portion of the bladder, and the diameter of the needle is quite small (3 to 5 mm), it has been our experience that continuous postoperative drainage is not required. In these situations, we proceed as we would if no perforation had occurred (i.e., the patient undergoes a voiding trial and if able to void successfully is sent home without a catheter). However, in certain situations, we would recommend drainage for a few days to a week (i.e., if multiple perforations occurred, if there is significant hematuria, or if the perforation was low in the base of the bladder).

Case 5: Excision of Suburethral Portion of Synthetic Sling and Partial Cystectomy to Remove Eroded Sling with Stone Formation from Bladder

 (Video 14-3)

A 67-year-old patient presents with a 4-year history of severe vaginal and pelvic pain. She underwent a TVT procedure approximately 6 years ago. She did very well for the first 2 years and then began to develop pain in her vagina and diffuse pelvic pain. She saw numerous physicians including multiple pain specialists, and no one could diagnosis the etiology of the pain. On examination, the pain is isolated in the distal left vaginal fornix in the area where the TVT is underneath the inferior pubic ramus on that side. She also complains of diffuse pelvic pain mostly on the left side. Cystoscopy reveals a 2 cm × 2 cm bladder stone attached to a small piece of the synthetic tape that was present in the bladder. The plan is to excise the suburethral part of the tape vaginally especially on the left side and perform an exploratory laparotomy with partial cystectomy to remove the tape and stone from the bladder.

Discussion of Case

Patients who present with vaginal or pelvic pain who have a history of any procedure for SUI should always undergo a thorough endoscopic evaluation of the urethra and bladder to rule out foreign body penetration or stone formation. Not performing this evaluation significantly delayed the diagnosis and created unwarranted prolonged pain in this patient.

Case 6: Excision of TVT-Secur Sling from Urethra with Urethral Reconstruction and Placement of Cadaveric Fascial Pubovaginal Sling

 (Video 14-4)

A 46-year-old woman who underwent a TVT-Secur (Ethicon, Somerville, NJ) procedure 1 year before presents with significant worsening of urinary leakage and de novo development of irritative symptoms including frequency, urgency, and dysuria. She had an injection of a bulking agent 9 months before presentation, which failed to improve her recurrent stress incontinence. On examination, she has obvious urethral hypermobility with some anterior vaginal wall descent and easily demonstrates the sign of SUI
with coughing in the supine position with a subjectively empty bladder. Cystourethroscopy demonstrates synthetic sling material present in the midportion of the lumen of the urethra. The patient subsequently underwent a vaginal excision of the TVT-Secur sling with a reconstruction of the urethra and placement of a cadaveric fascia lata pubovaginal sling. Postoperatively, the patient had continuous bladder drainage for 1 week and subsequently had resolution of SUI and significant improvement of irritative symptoms.

Discussion of Case

This case presents a situation in which the single-incision sling most likely was initially placed in the wall of the urethra. The surgeon dissected into a plane that was too deep and ended up placing the sling in the wall of the urethra. As discussed in Chapter 3, there is no clear plane of dissection between the distal anterior vaginal wall and the distal urethra. When initiating a vaginal incision for a MUS procedure, the surgeon needs to dissect well into the fibromuscular layer of the vaginal wall but stops short of the posterior wall of the urethra. In the authors' opinion, making the incision a bit larger and continuing the dissection lateral to the inferior pubic ramus facilitates dissection into this appropriate plane because it completely isolates and identifies the midportion of the urethra and the appropriate plane for sling placement. In this situation, the patient had recurrent SUI with synthetic sling material in her urethra. For this reason, we chose a biologic material to be used for a proximal pubovaginal sling. Placing another synthetic sling in a patient in whom it is known that an incision in the wall of the urethra is going to be made would be contraindicated because of concerns regarding breakdown of the urethral construction and the subsequent erosion of sling material back into the urethra.

Case 7: Complete Removal of Transobturator Tape (OB Tape) Secondary to Recurrent Granulation Tissue and Vaginal Bleeding

 (Video 14-5)

A 41-year-old woman has a history of placement of a transobturator sling (OB Tape; Mentor Urology, Santa Barbara, CA) approximately 2.5 years earlier. She subsequently experiences significant vaginal bleeding and recurrent granulation tissue. The suburethral part of the sling is removed, and later a second attempt is made to excise more granulation tissue because of persistent bleeding. When the patient comes for treatment, it is apparent that large areas of granulation tissue are still present, which indicates a continuous, ongoing inflammatory reaction between the sling material and the patient's tissue. The plan is to dissect into the obturator space and if necessary open up the inner thigh to remove the remaining mesh. The remainder of the sling was successfully removed via the vaginal route, and the vagina healed without incident.

Discussion of Case

A finding of persistent granulation tissue indicates the presence of an ongoing reaction between the foreign body and the surrounding tissue, and complete excision of the foreign body is usually required. This reaction generally occurs when non–type I macroporous mesh is used (as was the case with the OB Tape).

Case 8: Recurrent Incontinence After Tension-Free Vaginal Tape Secondary to Complex Urethral Diverticulum

 (Video 14-6)

A 61-year-old patient presents with persistent SUI after a TVT sling procedure performed approximately 6 weeks prior. Preoperative urodynamics studies noted evidence of urodynamic SUI with a stable bladder. She also developed de novo urgency and urge incontinence after placement of the TVT sling. Evaluation includes a repeat urodynamics study and cystourethroscopy. During urethroscopic examination, the patient is noted to have a large midurethral diverticulum. In view of these findings and the fact that she has developed de novo urgency and urge incontinence, it is decided to proceed with a takedown of the suburethral portion of the TVT sling in conjunction with a repair of the urethral diverticulum.

Discussion of Case

This case underscores the importance of a full evaluation, which should include cystourethroscopy, in a patient with recurrent or persistent incontinence after previous operation. Because repeat urodynamics studies showed persistent SUI, it could be argued that a repeat sling should be performed. However, if that would have occurred, the patient would have continued to leak because she was leaking secondary to overflow of urine from the urethral diverticulum during stress provocation.

Case 9: Excision of Eroded Tension-Free Vaginal Tape, with Repair of Urethrovaginal Fistula and Placement of Cadaveric Fascia Pubovaginal Sling

 (Video 14-7)

A 56-year-old patient presents 9 months after a retropubic synthetic sling procedure with severe recurrent SUI, erosion of the sling into the vaginal lumen, and a urethrovaginal fistula at the level of the midurethra. On examination, there is recurrent urethral incontinence that is stress related. Urodynamics notes stress incontinence at a volume of 200 mL in the sitting position with a Valsalva leak point pressure of 52 cm H_2O. Cystourethroscopy confirms the urethrovaginal fistula in the area of the midurethra. The patient underwent excision of the eroded synthetic sling with repair of the urethrovaginal fistula and placement of a cadaveric fascia pubovaginal sling.

Discussion of Case

This case describes a complication that most likely occurred because of an inappropriate anterior vaginal wall dissection leading to development of a urethrovaginal fistula and erosion of the synthetic sling. If the initial dissection is too deep, there is a chance of urethral injury with subsequent fistula formation or the potential for urethral erosion. There is no distinct plane of dissection between the distal anterior vaginal wall and posterior urethra. For this reason, sharp dissection must clearly separate these structures in an appropriate plane.

Case 10: Avoiding and Managing Bleeding During Placement of Retropubic Midurethral Sling

 (Video 14-8)

A 51-year-old woman undergoes an uncomplicated retropubic MUS procedure for SUI. She goes to the recovery area and begins to have mild tachycardia and some hypotension. Her preoperative hemoglobin was in the range of 12 g, postoperative hemoglobin is 8.0 g. The patient is examined and is noted to have a significant decrease in blood pressure when she sits up (orthostatic hypotension). Her abdomen is still soft, with adequate urine output. Blood type and screen is performed, and she is transfused with 2 units of blood and admitted to be observed overnight. Subsequent hemoglobin levels stabilize at 9.5 g, and a computed tomography scan is ordered at 6 AM the following day, which demonstrates an 8 cm × 10 cm retropubic hematoma. She is observed for the following 12 hours and again remains stable with a hemoglobin of approximately 10.0 g and stable vital signs. She is unable to void spontaneously and is discharged with a Foley catheter in place. There is spontaneous resolution of the retropubic hematoma over the upcoming 4 weeks. The patient is able to void spontaneously 2 weeks after her procedure.

Discussion of Case

The retropubic space has a very abundant blood supply. Numerous vessels can be injured during the blind passage of a retropubic MUS trocar, including the vessels in the wall of the vagina (veins of Santorini), aberrant obturator vessels, the obturator neurovascular bundle, and the external iliac and femoral vessels in rare cases. This case did not involve a major vessel injury, and for this reason it was reasonable to observe the hematoma and allow it to resolve spontaneously. Generally, the retropubic space is a very forgiving space, and these stable hematomas usually resolve without complications. However, in a patient whose condition does not stabilize with blood transfusion, one must consider a major vessel injury, which would either be the obturator neurovascular bundle or the external iliac or femoral vessels. In such a case, most likely exploratory laparotomy would be required. Also, one could consider an attempt at embolization of the bleeding vessel. See **Video 14-8** for discussion and demonstration of the various vessels that can be injured during retropubic MUS placement.

Case 11: Avoiding and Managing Small Bowel Injury During Placement of Retropubic Midurethral Sling

 (Video 14-9)

A 47-year-old woman undergoes a retropubic synthetic MUS procedure for SUI. Pertinent past medical history includes a ruptured appendix with acute peritonitis that occurred when she was a teenager. The procedure is believed to be uncomplicated, and the patient is discharged home with instructions to follow up in the office in 2 weeks. Approximately 12 hours after discharge, she complains of significant abdominal bloating, nausea, and vomiting. She presents to the emergency department, and her abdomen is noted to be quite distended with hypoactive bowel sounds. X-ray confirms free air in the abdomen. It is thought that a bowel injury occurred secondary to passage of the TVT needles. She undergoes exploratory laparotomy, and the sling is seen to be passing through a loop of small bowel that is firmly adhered in the lower pelvis. She undergoes a partial resection of the small bowel with removal of the TVT and recovers without incident.

Discussion of Case

Small bowel injury during retropubic MUS placement has been described. Before passage of trocars, patients should be placed in a mild Trendelenburg position (approximately 15 degrees), and in the authors' opinion, the procedure is probably best avoided in patients with a history of significant pelvic adhesions or peritonitis, as was the situation in this case. When patients develop abdominal distention, nausea, and signs of the small bowel obstruction postoperatively, one should always consider the possibility of injury to the small bowel.

Suggested Readings

Abdel-Fattah M, Ramsay I, Pringle S, et al. Evaluation of transobturator tension-free vaginal tapes in management of women with recurrent stress urinary incontinence. *Urology*. 2011;77:1070-1075.

Abrams P, Cardozo L, Fall M, et al. The standardization of terminology in lower urinary tract function: report from the standardization sub-committee of the International Continence Society. *Neurourol Urodyn*. 2002;21:167-178.

Albo ME, Richter HE, Brubaker L, et al. Burch colposuspension versus fascial sling to reduce urinary stress incontinence. *N Engl J Med*. 2007;356:2143-2155.

Amundsen CL, Flynn BJ, Webster GD. Anatomical correction of vaginal vault prolapse by uterosacral ligament fixation in women who also require a pubovaginal sling. *J Urol*. 2003;169:1770-1774.

Biggs GY, Ballert KN, Rosenblum N, et al. Patient-reported outcomes for tension-free vaginal tape-obturator in women treated with a previous anti-incontinence procedure. *Int Urogynecol J*. 2009;20:331-335.

Borstad E, Abdelnoor M, Staff AC, et al. Surgical strategies for women with pelvic organ prolapse and urinary stress incontinence. *Int Urogynecol J*. 2010;21:179-186.

Borstad E, Rud T. The risk of developing urinary stress incontinence after vaginal repair in continent women: a clinical and urodynamic follow-up study. *Acta Obstet Gynecol Scand*. 1989;68:545-549.

Botros SM, Miller JJ, Goldberg RP, et al. Detrusor overactivity and urge urinary incontinence following trans obturator versus midurethral slings. *Neurourol Urodyn*. 2007;26:42-45.

Casiano ER, Gebhart JB, McGree MM, et al. Does concomitant prolapse repair at the time of midurethral sling affect recurrent rates of incontinence? *Int Urogynecol J*. 2011;22:819-825.

Dmochowski RR, Blaivas JM, Gormley EA, et al. Update of AUA guideline on the surgical management of female stress urinary incontinence. *J Urol*. 2010;183:1906-1914.

Duckett JR, Tamilselvi A. Effect of tension-free vaginal tape in women with a urodynamic diagnosis of idiopathic detrusor overactivity and stress incontinence. *BJOG*. 2006;113:30-33.

Gamble T, Botros S, Beaumont J, et al. Predictors of persistent detrusor overactivity after transvaginal sling procedures. *Am J Obstet Gynecol*. 2008;199:696.e1-696.e7.

Groutz A, Blaivas JG, Hyman MJ, et al. Pubovaginal sling surgery for simple stress urinary incontinence: analysis by an outcome score. *J Urol*. 2001;165:1597-1600.

Holmgren C, Nilsson S, Lanner L, et al. Long-term results with tension-free vaginal tape on mixed and stress urinary incontinence. *Obstet Gynecol*. 2005;106:38-43.

Jain P, Jirschele K, Botros SM, et al. Effectiveness of midurethral slings in mixed urinary incontinence: a systematic review and meta-analysis. *Int Urogynecol J*. 2011;22:923-932.

Kulseng-Hanssen S, Husby H, Shiotz HA. Follow-up of TVT operations in 1,113 women with mixed urinary incontinence at 7 and 38 months. *Int Urogynecol J*. 2008;19:391-396.

Lee HN, Lee YS, Han JY, et al. Transurethral injection of bulking agent for treatment of failed midurethral sling procedures. *Int Urogynecol J*. 2010a;21:1479-1483.

Lee JH, Cho MC, Oh SJ, et al. Long-term outcome of the tension-free vaginal tape procedure in female urinary incontinence: a 6-year follow-up. *Korean J Urol*. 2010b;51:409-415.

Liapis A, Bakas P, Creatsas G. Tension-free vaginal tape in the management of recurrent urodynamic stress incontinence after previous failed midurethral tape. *Eur Urol*. 2009;55:1450-1458.

Long CY, Hsu SC, Wu TP, et al. Urodynamic comparison of continent and incontinent women with severe uterovaginal prolapse. *J Reprod Med*. 2004;49:33-37.

Mallet VT, Brubaker L, Stoddard AM, et al. The expectations of patients who undergo surgery for stress incontinence. *Am J Obstet Gynecol*. 2008;198:308.e1-308.e6.

Meltomaa S, Backman T, Haarala M. Concomitant vaginal surgery did not affect outcome of the tension-free vaginal tape operation during a prospective 3-year follow-up study. *J Urol*. 2004;172:222-226.

Ogah J, Cody JD, Rogerson L. Minimally invasive synthetic suburethral sling operations for stress urinary incontinence in women. *Cochrane Database Syst Rev*. 2009;(4):CD006375.

Paick JS, Oh SJ, Kim SW, Ku JH. Tension-free vaginal tape, suprapubic arc sling, and transobturator tape in the treatment of mixed urinary incontinence in women. *Int Urogynecol J*. 2008;19:391-396.

Petrou SP, Frank I. Complications and initial continence rates after a repeat pubovaginal sling procedure for recurrent stress urinary incontinence. *J Urol*. 2001;165:1979-1981.

Reena C, Kekre AN, Kekre N. Occult stress incontinence in women with pelvic organ prolapse. *Int J Obstet Gynecol*. 2007;97:31-34.

Sabadell J, Poza JL, Esgueva A, et al. Usefulness of retropubic tape for recurrent stress incontinence after transobturator tape failure. *Int Urogynecol J*. 2011;22(12):1543-1547.

Stav K, Dwyer PL, Rosamilia A, et al. Long-term outcomes of patients who failed to attend following midurethral sling surgery—a comparative study and analysis of risk factors for non-attendance. *Aust N Z J Obstet Gynaecol*. 2010;50:173-178.

Sze EHM, Kohli N, Miklos JR, et al. A retrospective comparison of abdominal sacrocolpopexy with Burch colposuspension versus sacrospinous fixation with transvaginal needle suspension for the management of vaginal vault prolapse and coexisting stress incontinence. *Int Urogynecol J.* 1999;10:390-393.

Togami JM, Chow D, Winters JC. To sling or not sling at the time of anterior vaginal compartment repair. *Curr Opin Urol.* 2010;20:269-274.

Wang F, Song Y, Huang H. Prospective randomized trial of TVT and TOT as primary treatment for female stress urinary incontinence with or without pelvic organ prolapse in southeast China. *Arch Gynecol Obstet.* 2010;281:279-286.

Sample Questionnaires and Symptom Measurement Tools for Women Complaining of Urinary Incontinence

Urogenital Distress Inventory-6 and Incontinence Impact Questionnaire -7

INCONTINENCE QUESTIONNAIRE (UDI-6)

DO YOU EXPERIENCE ANY URINARY INCONTINENCE? ____ YES _____ NO
Please circle the number that best describes what you are feeling.

Do you experience and, if so, how much are you bothered by:

	Not at all	Slightly	Moderately	Greatly
1. Frequent urination?	0	1	2	3
2. Urine leakage related to the feeling of urgency?	0	1	2	3
3. Urine leakage related to physical activity, coughing, or sneezing?	0	1	2	3
4. Small amounts of urine leakage?	0	1	2	3
5. Difficulty emptying your bladder?	0	1	2	3
6. Pain or discomfort in the lower abdomen or genital area?	0	1	2	3

INCONTINENCE IMPACT QUESTIONNAIRE- SHORT FORM IIQ-7

Some people find that accidental urine loss may affect their activities, relationships, and feelings. The questions below refer to areas in your life that may have been influenced or changed by your problem. For each question, circle the response that best describes how much your activities, relationships, and feelings are being affected by urine leakage.

Has urine leakage affected your...

	Not at all	Slightly	Moderately	Greatly
1. Ability to do household chores such as cooking, housecleaning, laundry?	0	1	2	3
2. Physical recreation such as walking, swimming, or other exercise?	0	1	2	3
3. Entertainment activities (movies, concerts, etc.)?	0	1	2	3
4. Ability to travel by car or bus more than 30 minutes from home?	0	1	2	3
5. Participation in social activities outside your home?	0	1	2	3
6. Emotional health (nervousness, depression, etc.)?	0	1	2	3
7. Feeling frustrated?	0	1	2	3

For both the UDI-6 and IIQ-7, obtain the mean value of all answered items (possible value 0-3), then multiply by 331/3 to obtain the scale score (range 0-100).

(From Ubersax JS, Wyman JF, Shumaker SA, et al. Short forms to assess life quality and symptom distress for urinary incontinence in women: the Incontinence Impact Questionnaire and the Urogenital Distress Inventory. Neurourol Urodyn. 1995;14:31.)

International Consultation on Incontinence Questionnaire-Short Form (ICIQ-SF)

ICIQ-SF

Many people leak urine some of the time. We are trying to find out how many people leak urine, and how much this bothers them. We would be grateful if you could answer the following questions, thinking about how you have been, on average, over the PAST FOUR WEEKS.

1. Please write in your date of birth:

☐☐ ☐☐ ☐☐
DAY   MONTH   YEAR

2. Are you (tick one):   Female ☐   Male ☐

3. How often do you leak urine? (Tick one box):

never	☐	0
about once a week or less often	☐	1
two or three times a week	☐	2
about once a day	☐	3
several times a day	☐	4
all the time	☐	5

4. We would like to know how much urine you think leaks. How much urine do you usually leak (whether you wear protection or not)? (Tick one box):

none	☐	0
a small amount	☐	2
a moderate amount	☐	4
a large amount	☐	5

5. Overall, how much does leaking urine interfere with your everyday life?
Please ring a number between 0 (not at all) and 10 (a great deal)

0   1   2   3   4   5   6   7   8   9   10
not at all   a great deal

ICIQ score: sum scores 3+4+5   ☐☐

6. When does urine leak? (Please tick all that apply to you)

never–urine does not leak ☐
leaks before you can get to the toilet ☐
leaks when you cough or sneeze ☐
leaks when you are asleep ☐
leaks when you are physically active/exercising ☐
leaks when you have finished urinating and are dressed ☐
leaks for no obvious reason ☐
leaks all the time ☐

Thank you very much for answering these questions.
Copyright © "ICIQ GROUP"

(From Avery K, Donovan J, Peters TJ, et al. ICIQ: a brief and robust measure for evaluating the symptoms and impact of urinary incontinence. Neurourol Urodyn. 2004;23:322.)

Incontinence Quality of Life Instrument (I-QOL)

Incontinence Quality of Life (I-QOL) Instrument

1. I worry about not being able to get to the toilet on time.
2. I worry about coughing or sneezing because of my urinary problems or incontinence.
3. I have to be careful standing up after I've been sitting down because of my urinary problems or incontinence.
4. I worry about where toilets are in new places.
5. I feel depressed because of my urinary problems or incontinence.
6. Because of my urinary problems or incontinence, I don't feel free to leave my home for long periods of time.
7. I feel frustrated because my urinary problems or incontinence prevents me from doing what I want.
8. I worry about others smelling urine on me.
9. Incontinence is always on my mind.
10. It's important for me to make frequent trips to the toilet.
11. Because of my urinary problems or incontinence, it's important to plan every detail in advance.
12. I worry about my urinary problems or incontinence getting worse as I grow older.
13. I have a hard time getting a good night of sleep because of my urinary problems or incontinence.
14. I worry about being embarrassed or humiliated because of my urinary problems or incontinence.
15. My urinary problems or incontinence makes me feel like I'm not a healthy person.
16. My urinary problems or incontinence makes me feel helpless.
17. I get less enjoyment out of life because of my urinary problems or incontinence.
18. I worry about wetting myself.
19. I feel like I have no control over my bladder.
20. I have to watch what or how much I drink because or my urinary problems or incontinence.
21. My urinary problems or incontinence limit my choice of clothing.
22. I worry about having sex because of my urinary problems or incontinence.

All items use the following response scale:

1 = Extremely
2 = Quite a bit
3 = Moderately
4 = A little
5 = Not at all

Subscale structure:

Avoidance and limiting behavior: items 1, 2, 3, 4, 10, 11, 13, and 20.
Psychosocial impacts: items 5, 6, 7, 9, 15, 16, 17, and 21.
Social embarrassment: items 8, 12, 14, 18, and 19.

(From Patrick DL, Martin ML, Bushnell DM, et al. Quality of life of women with urinary incontinence: further development of the incontinence quality of life instrument [I-QOL]. Urology. 199;53:71.)

Instructions: Please fill out the following questionnaires to the best of your ability.
If the question does not apply to you, please skip to the next question.

AUA SYMPTOM SCORE (AUASS)

Question: In the past month:	Not at all	Less than 1 time in 5	Less than half the time	About half the time	More than half the time	Almost always
How often have you had a sensation of not emptying your bladder completely after you finished urinating?	0	1	2	3	4	5
How often have you had to urinate again less than two hours after you finished urinating?	0	1	2	3	4	5
How often have you found you stopped and started again several times when you urinated?	0	1	2	3	4	5
How often have you found it difficult to postpone urination?	0	1	2	3	4	5
How often have you had a weak urinary stream?	0	1	2	3	4	5
How often have you had to push or strain to begin urination?	0	1	2	3	4	5
	None	1 time	2 times	3 times	4 times	5 or more times
How many times per night did you most typically get up to urinate from the time you went to bed at night until the time you got up in the morning?	0	1	2	3	4	5

QUALITY OF LIFE (QoL)

Question:	Delighted	Pleased	Mostly satisfied	Mixed	Mostly dissatisfied	Unhappy	Terrible
If you were to spend the rest of your life with your urinary condition just the way it is now, how would you feel about that?	0	1	2	3	4	5	6

Index

Page numbers followed by "f" indicate figures, and "t" indicate tables.

Printed and bound by CPI Group (UK) Ltd, Croydon, CR0 4YY

08/05/2025

01864793-0001

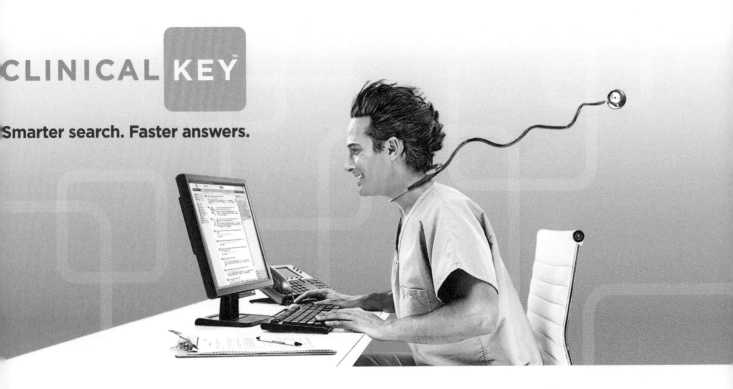